HEROIC ACTS
in Humble Shoes
America's Nurses Tell Their Stories

Pat —
To your heroic work.
It was wonderful meeting you
today! Best,
Irene 5/11

HEROIC ACTS
in Humble Shoes

America's Nurses Tell Their Stories

Irene Stemler, RN, BSN

Irene Stemler.

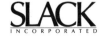

SLACK

INCORPORATED

www.slackbooks.com

ISBN: 978-1-55642-904-0

Copyright © 2009 by SLACK Incorporated

Cover photo: Irene Stemler
Cover design: Nadine Kost

The procedures and practices described in this book should be implemented in a manner consistent with the professional standards set for the circumstances that apply in each specific situation. Every effort has been made to confirm the accuracy of the information presented and to correctly relate generally accepted practices. The authors, editor, and publisher cannot accept responsibility for errors or exclusions or for the outcome of the material presented herein. There is no expressed or implied warranty of this book or information imparted by it. Care has been taken to ensure that drug selection and dosages are in accordance with currently accepted/recommended practice. Due to continuing research, changes in government policy and regulations, and various effects of drug reactions and interactions, it is recommended that the reader carefully review all materials and literature provided for each drug, especially those that are new or not frequently used. Any review or mention of specific companies or products is not intended as an endorsement by the author or publisher.

SLACK Incorporated uses a review process to evaluate submitted material. Prior to publication, educators or clinicians provide important feedback on the content that we publish. We welcome feedback on this work.

Published by: SLACK Incorporated
                       6900 Grove Road
                       Thorofare, NJ 08086 USA
                       Telephone: 856-848-1000
                       Fax: 856-848-6091
                       www.slackbooks.com

Contact SLACK Incorporated for more information about other books in this field or about the availability of our books from distributors outside the United States.

Library of Congress Cataloging-in-Publication Data
Heroic acts in humble shoes : America's nurses tell their stories / [edited by] Irene Stemler.
     p. ; cm.
  ISBN 978-1-55642-904-0
1. Nursing--United States. I. Stemler, Irene
  [DNLM: 1. Nurses--United States--Personal Narratives. 2. Nursing--United States--Personal Narratives. WZ 112.5.N8 H559 2009]
  RT4.H47 2009
  610.73--dc22

                                        2009016259

Printed in the United States of America.

Last digit is print number: 10   9   8   7   6   5   4   3   2   1

Dedication

To my Grandfather—a shoemaker

Contents

Acknowledgments

There have been so many people who have left their mark on this project, and I am deeply grateful to each and every one. I've always thought of myself as a lucky person, which doesn't necessarily equate to wealth and splendor in a material sense, but it does in terms of richness of experiences and being surrounded by loving friends and family. Thank you for your support, encouragement, and generosity of spirit.

The following people have contributed more than they will know, at crucial points in this journey. Laura Bailey, Eileen Hurn, Ausra Kiela, Susan Klein Weiner, Jim LaFrancis, Kurt Meyer, Cindy Thelen, and David Vick have known me the longest and have always supported me in all of my work. I would like to thank you from the bottom of my heart for your unwavering friendship, days of endless discussions, and late nights of napkin diagrams imagining the perfect nursing shoes display.

Tom Koppes and Linda Polzin are 2 of the best nurses I will ever know. Thank you for your critical eye and keeping me grounded while editing these interviews.

To Jennifer Ferris of Kelsey Transcripts, thank you for taking on the daunting task of transcribing hundreds of hours of audio tape.

This project would have never taken on this form if not for an art exhibition at Patrick Hilton's Exurbia Gallery where John Tolley and Randy Vick were showing their latest work. Thank you for sparking the creative potential for a quirky exhibit of used nursing shoes and the stories behind them! I'd also like to extend my sincere appreciation to John Bond and the editors at SLACK Incorporated for helping make this book a reality. It has been a true collaboration from the start.

Every new idea needs a fertile place to grow and I'd like to thank Susan McBroom for referring me to authors and engaging in philosophical discussions that allowed me to view health care and nursing practice in a different way. I'd also like to thank my friends in The Chapter Four Society and the WOTOP Group for their positive thoughts and encouragement.

The last leg of the writing process has been an interesting and tumultuous time, and I have to thank my brother and sister-in-law, Andy and Nikki Stemler, and my mom, Mary Stemler, for their love and understanding. Lola found a comfy spot and stationed herself at my computer during long nights of writing, and Brandi was present during every interview.

I would especially like to thank my friend and mentor, Deb Gauldin. If we could harness the laughter we've enjoyed throughout the years, and share it with our neighbors, the world would be a better place.

Lastly, I would like to acknowledge the special group of nurses who agreed to be interviewed for this project. If we could clone you, we'd be able to put an end to our nursing shortage and health care crisis. I'm a lucky person—I managed to find just the right blend of powerful, intelligent, humorous, and compassionate nurses, and encouraged them to tell their stories. Thank you all.

I would like to acknowledge the following individuals for permission to reprint the following material:

"Culpae." Reprinted by permission of Carol Battaglia. Excerpted from the book *Drifting Among the Whales*, published by Vista Publishing. © 1999 Carol Battaglia.

Unsung Heroes. Reprinted by permission of Deb Gauldin Productions, Inc. © 2004 Deb Gauldin and Irene Stemler.

Photo of Jo Groves taken by Mark Fredericks and used with permission.
Photo of Marian Tylk taken by Linda Polzin and used with permission.
Photo of Irene Stemler taken by David Vick and used with permission.

The following interviews faithfully represent the conversations I had with the nurses I interviewed. For the sake of clarity, I made some grammatical changes and other edits.

About the Author

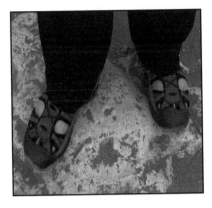

Irene Stemler is a registered nurse and holds a bachelor's degree in Nursing from Rush University in Chicago. She has more than 20 years of health care experience in nursing management, education, advocacy, and consulting. Irene had been working on a federally funded nurse retention grant at the University of Illinois, and most recently has been focusing on nurse recruitment strategies for the federal government. She is a former vice president of clinical services for a national assisted living company where she co-developed the corporation's signature health and wellness program. Irene has worked with a variety of health care organizations in the areas of clinical program development, regulatory compliance, case management, staff development, and marketing.

While a lifelong Chicagoan (Sox over Cubs), her career has offered her a tremendous opportunity to travel the country and present at numerous conferences on issues central to nurse recruitment and retention. Her most meaningful improvisational lesson learned while a student at The Second City was the concept of "Yes, and..." which is to accept whatever's given and give back something of equal or greater value. This concept is evidenced by her work in nursing recognition. A published author of stories on nursing, Irene is also the creator of *Heroic Acts in Humble Shoes: America's Nurses Tell Their Stories,* a traveling exhibit of well-worn nursing shoes and the stories of the nurses who wear them.

The exhibition became the inspiration for this book—a diverse collection of stories that celebrates and honors nurses from all backgrounds and areas of expertise. Her work with health care organizations uses aspects of storytelling in building strong teams and developing effective leaders.

Preface

This book gives voice to the millions of nurses who are providing compassionate care in the face of unprecedented challenges to our health care system. *Heroic Acts in Humble Shoes: America's Nurses Tell Their Stories* is like *Chicken Soup for the Soul* meets *SiCKO*.

This book contains interviews with nurses from across the country, and each story opens with a photo of the nurse's shoes. You'll be surprised at what you see, and read. These well-worn nursing shoes and intimate, passionate stories bring well-deserved recognition and much needed inspiration to millions of nurses in this country, not to mention the many millions more who come in contact with nurses each day.

Chances are you know a nurse. There might be one in your family, you live next door to one, or a nurse has taken care of you or someone you love. Chances are, you don't know about a potentially catastrophic global nursing shortage that will change health care delivery.

The United States is in the midst of a global health care crisis, which hinges on these simple truths:

- Nurse vacancy rates in hospitals and clinics have reached an all-time high, and continue to soar at alarming speed.
- Patients in hospitals with the highest patient-to-nurse ratio (8 patients per nurse) have a 31% greater risk of dying than those in hospitals with 4 patients per nurse.
- There are not enough nursing instructors to accommodate the numbers of students interested in applying to schools of nursing.
- There is a general lack of understanding in government and the public of the vital role that nurses play in health care delivery.

This book explores the deepest core of health care, the relationship between the nurse and the patient. It reveals what nurses truly endure as they battle to provide quality health care to ordinary people on a daily basis. It dispels the myth that nurses are sex symbols, Nurse Ratcheds, or physician's handmaids. Through this collection of intimate stories and eclectic display of nursing shoes, the reader will know that nurses have one thing in common: the desire to provide compassionate care on their terms.

Since the days of Florence Nightingale and her pioneering work on the battlefields in the Crimean War, nursing has come to play a significant role in times of military conflict—at home and abroad. Today, nurses are volunteering to support our men and women in the Middle East; taking on tremendously dangerous assignments that test the meaning of the word "heroic." At home, nurses are diligently preparing for terrorist attacks or natural disasters and learning to become "first responders" in times of crisis. It's a much different battlefield today.

Heroic Acts in Humble Shoes also provides a springboard for spirited discussion about the future of nursing and health care in this country. It should be used not only in the classroom setting, encouraging discussions on ethics and leadership, but it should also be found in Congress and in the Senate. Legislators would be wise to refer to individual stories to support their cases for improved funding for schools of nursing.

In an age of rising health care costs, associated primarily with treating increasing numbers of uninsured patients and being dictated to by HMOs, nurses are the ones who have shouldered the burden—by enduring staffing cuts and accepting noncompetitive salaries.

In the end nurses are overworked and undervalued, and patients are the ones who pay—in some cases, with their lives. As the patient-to-nurse ratios rise, unsafe working conditions emerge, regardless of the qualifications of the nurse. Many nurses are being driven from the bedside because they can no longer provide skilled, compassionate care in a safe working environment, not with short-staffing and mandatory overtime. The ones who remain should be honored for their heroic work on yet another battlefield.

Heroic Acts in Humble Shoes marks a turning point in nursing. When nurses read these stories and visions for the future, they'll be encouraged to take a leadership position in transforming their profession and nurses' role in health care delivery.

We speak of power in nursing, but we can't address our power until we are clear about our identity. Who are we as a profession, and what do we offer? What would we like to improve? What is nursing's future story? We have the ability to write it now; we simply need the wisdom and courage as a unified group to take our place at the table and lead that discussion.

Foreword

When I read the title of this book, at first I found myself thinking about the phrase "heroic acts" and wondering how I would apply it to nursing. Certainly I didn't think of acts of great courage or self-sacrifice, although many nurses are heroic in this way. But the more subtle meanings rang true for me: acts of great intensity, actions with powerful effect, understanding what must be done to keep others safe, and doing it, regardless of circumstance or consequence. Those words describe nursing at its core, and nurses who are passionate about their work know this to be true, without question... even if they don't say it out loud.

The stories in this book are the stories of nurses like that. For them, nursing is an art form and a learned practice, based in science and life wisdom. And because they practice nursing in this way, they change the world for the better, one life at a time, and mostly they don't care if anyone else notices.

Some do notice, of course. A wise and thoughtful man who survived a grave illness began directing his personal philanthropy to a school of nursing because, in his words, "People take nursing for granted. They don't give nurses nearly enough credit; they don't support nursing education or nursing research. When I was so ill in the hospital, without question, the physicians saved my life, and for that I am forever grateful. But they played no significant part in my recovery—and what good is saving my life if I do not recover my life? Nurses brought me back to my life. Nurses gave my life back to me."

This man understands the significance of nursing, as do many others whose lives were changed—whose lives were given back to them— by nurses. But the fact is that many others do not. They see nurses as assistants to physicians, or as technical workers responsible for a set of mundane tasks. At best, they see nursing as the consolation prize for those not smart enough for medical school; at worst, they see nursing as a necessary, but acutely embarrassing, variation on the theme that "a woman's place is in the home."

The folks who do understand the importance of nursing probably outnumber those who don't by a wide margin. Unfortunately, the damage done by negative stereotypes and demeaning attitudes about nursing has taken its toll: dramatic declines in nursing school enrollments in the 1980s and 90s, shockingly little public investment in nursing education and research, compared to that devoted to medical education and medical research, even in the face of the worst shortage in modern history, and now the vanishingly small number of nurses in positions of influence across the country, despite the fact that nothing in health care happens without nurses. As one nurse in this book points out, it is still too often true that when a patient receives excellent hospital care, the physician gets an endowed chair, and the nurses get candy and flowers.

This book can help change that. These stories are testimony to the difference nurses make every day—by understanding what must be done to keep others safe and doing it regardless of circumstance or consequence, and through countless acts of intensity and powerful effect that largely go unnoticed—by bringing people back to their lives.

Katharyn A. May, DNSc, RN, FAAN
Dean and Professor
University of Wisconsin–Madison
School of Nursing

Introduction

I've always loved listening to stories. My earliest recollection is of my grandmother telling me elaborate stories about Baba Yaga—old witch lore in the Polish tradition. What I didn't hear were stories about her life in Poland, and I knew nothing of my grandfather, who died in WWII.

Nearly 2 years after I began my work collecting nurses' shoes and their stories, I stumbled across a family story that would change my life. I learned that after my grandparents had married, they moved to my grandmother's farm. My grandfather was from the city and working on a farm was a very new experience for him. He wasn't very handy, but he kept himself busy in other ways.

The story could have ended there, but I asked a simple question, "What was his profession when he lived in the city?" The response? He was a cobbler—a shoemaker!

My work took on another, deeper meaning that day. I realized that a pair of worn nurse's shoes was the perfect symbol for a profession that needed mending—and that a shoemaker's granddaughter might be the ideal person to take up the cause.

I realized too, that the simple telling of a story, guided by a few thoughtful questions, holds incredible power—enough to influence one life and, hopefully, an entire profession.

What stories are you holding dear? I encourage you to share them.

SECTION ONE

"There is a certain embarrassment about being a storyteller in these times when stories are considered not quite as satisfying as statements and statements not quite as satisfying as statistics; but in the long run, a people is known, not by its statements or its statistics, but by the stories it tells."

Flannery O'Connor
"Mystery and Manners"

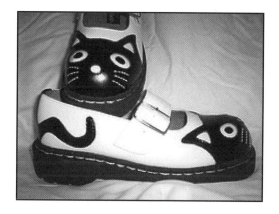

CHAPTER 1

Perfect Score

I have a degree in music because my dad wanted a musician in the family, even though I was good in math and science and wanted to go to medical school or be a biologist. In school I kept up my interest in science and added a major in sociology, and once I graduated I did everything in the world for 10 minutes at a time.

But I kept coming back to medical and scientific work. I ended up working at Planned Parenthood, and one of the nurse practitioners encouraged me to go into nursing. I took her advice and went back to nursing school, thinking I would eventually work in Women's Health.

After graduating, on a total lark, I interviewed at UT Southwestern University Hospital–Zale Lipshy, which is where I still work today. They offered me the job before I even left the interview. It was amazing. They apparently saw something I didn't and they knew it would be a good fit. They put me on the neuroscience floor, and I was immediately fascinated. Every single patient is different. The nice thing with neuroscience is that if there is something wrong with a person's brain or spine, you can see it immediately on the outside of their body. So it is good for somebody like me who has a short attention span. It's not like cardiology where you actually have to concentrate [laughs].

I was very fortunate to find an excellent situation right off. I know it sounds cliché, but the hospital system I work for is truly committed to patient care. Speaking for my unit, they make sure that the nurses are "partners" with the patients, so you don't get bombarded with a huge patient load.

We see neurologically impaired patients that no one else can diagnose. We admit patients from as far away as North Dakota to Arizona and Arkansas. Aside from the National Jewish Health in Colorado, we are the only research hospital in this region.

How long have you been a nurse?

Six years.

Do you see yourself doing this for 6 more?

Absolutely. I won't say that it's not frustrating because any kind of nursing is frustrating. But it is so interesting. There have been so many changes in nursing, and so much progress made in the field of neuroscience in particular, that I could easily see myself doing this for 20 years.

I'm very lucky to work with a really dedicated, really smart group of people, and we're in it because we like it and because we have fun. The people I work with have had the experience of being the smartest person in the room, and now they have to share that title. There's always someone who has more information and there's always something to learn here.

The hospital also values nurses. The attending physicians understand nurses are their eyes, ears, and noses on the floor. If an attending hears a resident being nasty to a nurse, she or he will take that resident aside and say that is not acceptable.

How do you develop a culture like that?

I think it's the longevity of the people who work here. The shortest tenure is about 2 years, which is very unusual, especially considering Texas is experiencing a huge nursing shortage. You have nurses coming in and getting their sign-on bonuses of $5,000 or more, and leaving 6 months later. That's how they supplement their income. The second thing is that the attending physicians we work with recognize that they can't get their work done without us and there is an astonishing lack of ego, even working with neurosurgeons. The neurosurgeons at Zale are good enough that they don't have to prove anything.

What are some of your success stories?

We had one really fantastic success with a young woman in her early twenties who suffered a grade 4 intracranial hemorrhage. She had a congenital aneurysm rupture. The prognosis for a grade 4 bleed is extremely poor, but she hung on and was on our floor for about 6 months. Then she went to rehab for another several months.

About a year and a half after being admitted she came back to the hospital and got married in the family room of our rehab unit. Our chaplain performed the ceremony and she was able to walk, unassisted, down the aisle.

That was huge because we didn't think she was going to make it out of ICU! People came in on their days off just to come to the wedding. It was amazing. Everybody felt like she was part of the family. She's living independently now and taking care of her child.

Do you ever process with the team what you've gone through with these patients?

I think there's a certain amount of distance that you have to achieve when you know somebody is going bad. But at the same time, when your colleague has a particularly difficult code, then we'll all make time to sit down and talk about it. And of course we have a chaplain and we have the doctors to talk to. When it's a situation where a patient dies shortly after being admitted, the processing is very personal because there is a certain amount of "anti-touchy-feely" among surgeons in general, and neurosurgeons in particular. If you get too invested in the process of grieving the patient, it makes you paranoid for the next person and that can be counterproductive.

Do you find that you're appreciated by your patients and their family members?

Yes.

Okay—you didn't even pause.

Patients thank me every day. My primary job is to educate my patients and to translate what the doctors tell them into English, and to reassure them that although this is their brain and this is scary, we do it hundreds if not thousands of times a year. Therefore, we will be on the lookout for anything that might go wrong. And every day I have somebody tell me, "Nobody has explained this as well as you have," or, "Thank you so much, I'm not as frightened now."

The best thank you I ever received was a complete surprise and arrived in person. I had a patient who was very, very sick with a central nervous system cancer. We decided it was in her best interest to transfer her to a hospital in Utah that specialized in this very tiny specialty of CNS cancer.

She walked back onto our unit about 6 months later, cured.

I cried when she showed up because I really didn't think that she'd live to see Utah. She made the trip back to Texas to thank us and she sought me out, in particular. I just broke down – with relief and in amazement that she was alive.

Because of the shortage of nurses some US hospitals have been involved in global recruitment efforts. I wonder if instead, perhaps we should start from scratch

and look at our own health care system and redefine nursing's role in that system.

Let me share a story that might illustrate your point. I recently adopted a dog and the woman who facilitated it was delighted that I was a nurse. She told me, "Oh, I don't need your paperwork, you're a nurse! I can trust you. I don't have to look at your house or your yard, and I know you'll take good care of him." That's the upside. We're the most trusted profession around. The downside is that instead of being seen as primarily scientists and educators, we're seen as bedpan pushers and helpmeets.

There are a lot of very bright, very assertive, and very tough young women and men who don't want to go into nursing because they see it as a secondary role. They don't see it as a profession equal to that of medicine. The doctors I work with are my colleagues. I'm not subservient; I'm not subsidiary. I have my own science that I practice and they have theirs and our two sciences are complementary. We need to make a big noise about that. If you want to get hands-on with patients, don't be a doctor, be a nurse.

When people ask me, "Why didn't you go to medical school? You're too smart to be a nurse." I always reply, "Do you want somebody stupid at your bedside?" "Do you want somebody stupid doing all the work?"

This is why I am astounded by the Joint Commission on the Accreditation of Healthcare Organizations (JCAHO) regulation that says doctors can no longer write range orders. For example, a pain medication order used to read, "… give 2 mg to 4 mg every 4 hours for pain." Now, the doctor has to write, "… 2 mg every 4 hours for mild pain, 1-4 on a scale of 1-10. And 4 mg every 4 hours for severe pain, 5-10 on a scale of 1-10."

Basically, they've taken away our brains. They have completely reversed what nurses have been fighting for, which is the ability to use our own clinical judgment, and capability for critical thinking. On a macro level we need to fight that kind of change because it's not a safety issue. That's a clinical judgment issue. Nurses are not prescribing; we're simply using clinical judgment and we need to make sure that clinical judgment is a component of patient safety. Patient safety can't happen without my trained clinical judgment and you need to acknowledge that as an organization.

By that simple act coming down under the guise of patient safety, it has moved us, in the minds of the largest health care accreditation group, from trained professionals to pill pushers.

If you had to describe what I do in one word it is "gatekeeper." And I am not the only gatekeeper, I have doctors and pharmacists and techs working with me who are better at certain things than I am, they notice things that I don't, and they have knowledge bases that I don't have. But at the end of the day I'm the one who has to assimilate this information. I have to qualify it and quantify it and put it into a framework that is easily understandable for every member of the health care team.

Any person on that team who has a question, whether it's the radiologist, pharmacist, doctor, or physical therapist, is going to come to the nurse because the nurse is expected to have a global view of the patient. We have to get the message across that this is what we do, and it is both intellectually and emotionally challenging. Our work is equal in value to the work of doctors and everybody else.

This is slightly off-topic, but there has been some discussion recently about professional appearance and styles of nursing uniforms. Do you have an opinion on that?

Honestly, I don't think bringing back a uniform is going to help. It's a romantic idea that you should be able to identify your nurse as the Angel in White, Seal Blue, or Hunter Green. Having a uniform to identify us will not make us any more professional until we redefine publicly and loudly what our professional capabilities and duties are. It doesn't matter what the uniform is until you change the story behind it. In other words, just having a uniform is not going to make us more professional because we haven't done a very good job articulating what our profession is.

Do you consider your work to be heroic?

[Long pause...] There's a writer named Ellis Peters who wrote a series of books involving a medieval monk called Brother Cadfael. He was essentially the 13th century Quincy. Her books deal with Cadfael's personality because he was a warrior for 40 years before he became a monk. One of her books has him reflecting that the step from ordinary to miraculous is so small that if you weren't paying attention you would miss it.

My work is heroic but it's heroic only in that the step from ordinary to heroic is so small. It is the tiniest difference in the things that I do and the way that I do them that makes my work heroic, and you would miss it if you weren't paying attention.

It really is as simple as tucking somebody in to make sure they're warm, because that's what they remember. At the end of the day nurses are the ones who are there for the patients. It is so easy to walk out of the room, and the fact that you stay makes a huge difference. I enjoy exercising my brain and I enjoy getting my dander up and solving problems, but I also enjoy the very small touches that make somebody feel better or make them feel safe.

I don't mean this in an arrogant way but there is a lot of power in nursing. It's a power that you should respect and learn to wield very carefully. But there are also a lot of very small, intimate touches that come from helping people to heal, and that is what keeps me coming back day after day.

That, and the fact that I can tell when someone is neurologically intact when they look down at my feet and say, "Is that a cat on your shoe?"

"Yes!" I shout. "Perfect score! Fifteen points on the Glasgow Coma Scale!"

Jo, RN
Staff Nurse, Neuroscience Unit
Texas

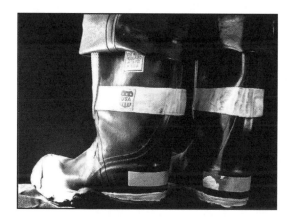

CHAPTER 2

First In

When I was growing up in Scotland there were no paramedics, and firemen didn't have any status at all. I studied chemistry with plans of becoming an industrial chemist, but I changed my focus and became a police officer. I worked in Edinburgh for a few years before moving to this country.

What led you to become a firefighter/paramedic?

This is a great story. When I came over here I drove a bus for a while, I pumped gas, I worked in construction, and for a surveying company. I was trying to figure out what I wanted to do with my life. When I was working construction, I met a great guy who worked for us 2 days a week. I asked him what he did on the other days, and he told me he was a firefighter.

One day he showed up at the worksite and said, "Here, fill this out. You should be a fireman." He had picked up the application for me, and even paid the fee. You know, I still owe him $20.

I've been a firefighter/paramedic for 13 years, and for the last 6 years I have also worked as a paramedic tech in the ER. My whole life has been focused on emergency medicine, and I felt that the natural progression would be to go into nursing. I thought about going on for my baccalaureate degree in fire science, but that only prepares you to be a fire chief. I would miss not being in the front lines. I like being first in—not knowing what to expect.

But isn't it unnerving to always approach the unknown?

None of us really feels that way. It's a huge adrenaline rush, but you also have the satisfaction of knowing that you have helped someone. You're the first one there and you're the one making decisions. When you walk in the door, people look at you and say, "I'm so glad you're here. Please help me." And then you go to work.

I also like the fast-paced setting of the ER, so I'll continue there as a nurse. I like thinking on my feet and making decisions.

In any of your roles, as a firefighter, paramedic, or nurse, have you ever considered your actions to be heroic?

No. It's my job. Somebody's got to do it, even though a lot of people tell me they couldn't do my job. There is never a day when I say that I don't want to go to work. A lieutenant at the fire station likes to say that if you really like your job, you'll never work another day in your life. You'll have so much fun that it's not considered work.

Do you think you've made the right choices regarding your career?

When I was growing up, I knew that I wanted to do something with my life. When I first came to this country and was interviewing for different jobs, I met an employer who asked me what I wanted out of life. I told him that I wanted my daughter to be proud of me. I wanted my daughter to grow up and say, "My dad is...this."

"So, you want a title," he said.

But I didn't want a title. I wanted to be something that she could be proud of, and that I am proud of. And she is proud. I'm a firefighter, a paramedic, and a nurse. It doesn't get any better than that. It really doesn't.

Colin Finlay, RN, EMT-P
Firefighter/Paramedic
Staff Nurse, Emergency Department
Illinois

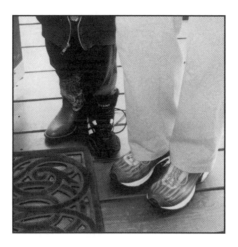

CHAPTER 3

Just the Basics

I have always loved teaching, and thought I would be a teacher forever. I actually taught first grade for 1 year, but the classroom situation was overwhelming. Eventually I went back to school and earned a degree in nursing.

I have been a rehab nurse for 17 years. I was always intrigued by emergency and intensive care nurses, but I knew that I wasn't going to be a "life-saver." That is the beauty of nursing. It fits all personalities.

I have a real appreciation for rehab nursing. I have the patience for it. I can remember my first day on the unit, and I was taking a patient to the bathroom. It took 15 minutes! But that is the essence of rehab nursing. It's not about hurrying to get to the next patient. It is about giving this patient the opportunity to stand up… pivot… remind him to move his right foot… reach for the bar… and so on. This is why they are in rehabilitation. They are re-learning the basics of self-care. This is the side of nursing that is not so hurried and fast paced. It's refreshing. There is actual time for teaching the patient and the family. Ideally, nursing is coupled with teaching.

Have you seen the Johnson & Johnson commercials?

Yes. Finally, there is public recognition for nursing! My boys were watching the commercial during the Olympics and my oldest turned to me and said, "Mommy, that's what you do. You're a nurse." I'm very proud of that.

Would you consider any of your actions or interventions to be heroic?

I really think that helping patients take those small steps are big steps for the patient. That's heroic for me. To help them feel good about themselves.

Christine Tolley, RN, CRRN
Registry Nurse, Rehabilitation
Illinois

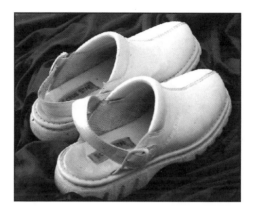

CHAPTER 4

My Mother's Gift

I always knew that I'd be a nurse. I started as a nurse's aide in the ER and continued there when I graduated and became a registered nurse. I've also been very involved in hospice care. People are amazed because they think these 2 areas are at opposite ends of the spectrum. In some ways they are right, but hospice care is also intense work. It is crisis management.

What makes you so passionate about end-of-life care?

I was taught by a great teacher. When my mom died of cancer she taught me how to die, so I wasn't afraid of it. A lot of people are afraid of that last breath, of being with a person in those last moments. It's one of the greatest transitions we make in our lives, and people want to know about it but they are afraid to ask. I am willing to teach them.

At one point during my mother's illness I needed to take her to the ER, and the first thing the resident wanted to know was her DNR (Do Not Resuscitate) status. Well, the oncologist never even broached the subject with us. We were totally into treatment and therapy. I had no idea, and told him that he would have to ask my mother what she wanted.

After what felt like an hour, I walked into her room and asked her what happened. "The doctor just wanted to know what I wanted to do if my heart stopped beating or I stopped breathing," she explained calmly from her hospital bed.

How did your mom answer that question?

She said, "Eileen, I really love you. I love dad and the boys, and I love my life here, but I'm also excited about meeting my maker. And when it comes time for me to do that, I don't want anything to artificially keep me from that experience."

I was crying at this point, and then she looked at me and said, "But I'm not dying yet." And she was right.

Six months later, she had a beautiful death. It's supposed to be a spiritual experience.

Eileen Hurn, RN, MS
Nurse Educator
Florida

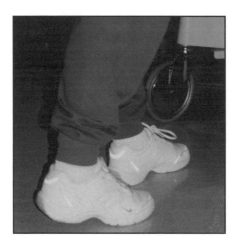

CHAPTER 5

High Tech—High Touch

"**H**ello. My name is Pam and I'll be taking care of you and your family tonight."

That is how I usually greet my patients in the ICU. If the patient is non-responsive, I usually have more interaction with the patient's close friends or relatives. Many times I'm not only taking care of the patient, but I'm also ministering to the family.

Patients in this unit are almost always there unwillingly. They have been thrown into these situations because of surgery, trauma, stroke, or heart attack. They are connected to so many machines and they have lost control of so many functions, that they have lost their dignity as well. I feel that as an intensive care nurse, it is my duty and obligation to help them through that emotional upheaval.

What gives you the greatest sense of satisfaction at work?

I enjoy taking care of people. I especially enjoy older people because I love to listen to their stories. I have a great respect for them and what they've lived through. I find it personally rewarding to take care of this population.

There are times when intensive care nurses get pegged as being more high-tech than high-touch. How would you respond to that?

Oh, I certainly get a rush from participating in emergency situations, but what stands out for me is simply being there for my patient. I remember when a nurse friend of mine was with a dying patient in the ICU. It was the patient's 53rd wedding anniversary and her husband was with her. My friend just sat there, holding the husband's hand while he wept.

Even though it's the ICU and you're not literally saving a life, you can still make a difference in someone's life. That makes work meaningful.

Pam DeFrancisco, RN
Staff Nurse, ICU
Illinois

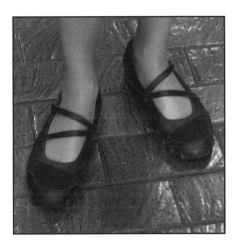

CHAPTER 6

Paradigm Shift

I am the dean of nursing in a health science university. Part of my not having any fanfare is because I'm part of a university that has a medical school and a veterinary college, and they're considered more "glitzy" than nursing. You can never win. If you're in nursing education in a liberal arts university they think you're a square peg in a round hole. Then you go to a health science university and nursing is still the square peg in a round hole. I was in a California State University, and they thought nursing was too expensive. Nursing education, no matter where you sit, at least in my experience, is not looked upon favorably.

Taking a step back, how did you become a nurse?

Actually, I didn't have any plan to be a nurse. I started out as a biology major with a psychology minor, which is what I thought I was going to do. A friend of mine said, "I'm going to a 4-year BSN program." I said, "Oh, really?" I just didn't know that you could get an RN degree at a 4-year university, but it just clicked. What a perfect blend of science and psychology. Then, on my very first day of orientation at San Francisco State University School of Nursing, it became clear that I wanted to be an educator.

The chair of the department was Reba de Tornyay, PhD, a well-known leader in nursing, and it just came together for me. Through my experience as a student I came to admire the faculty members who had a strong clinical background, and I told myself that I needed to work 10 years to be a clinical expert before becoming an educator. It was my divine plan from practically the first week of nursing school. It was absolutely clear to me, and after that I did everything along the way to make it happen.

I was very fortunate. The school followed a traditional calendar, so I worked every summer at a hospital, which has the same fine reputation today as it did when I worked there. I had more clinical experience than the average BSN nurse. Actually, in my senior year, I got fed up with the senior seminar because I was told, "You really should conduct patient care conferences on your units." I became frustrated as I was not gaining any skills to work in the real world. Instead, I said, "Unless you're going to teach me how this is relevant to the real work environment, I can't attend. We can't have care conferences when you have 1.5 LVNs based on the census. This is not reality."

I stomped out and was going to quit school, but one of the faculty members that facilitated that senior seminar came to me and said, "You can't quit. You're just the kind of nurse we need." She pulled me back, but I really almost dropped out. I felt like they were creating too much of a disconnect with the real world. She said, "No, you have to stick with it."

Her other pearl of wisdom to me was, "Do not ever leave a position without expressing why you are leaving. If you walk out and don't tell them why you are leaving, then you will never make change in that organization." And that is exactly what I have done. Even if I worked in a place that wasn't great, I would express why I was leaving to try to make it better. She really was a mentor, but I didn't see it at the time. When you are 21 you think you know everything.

Have you ever had a similar conversation with one of your own students?

I did. She's graduating this year. She was creating problems in her first semester and I actually had to write a memo to her file. It was embarrassing, but she wouldn't stop talking in the classroom. The faculty member had tried to explain to her that she was disrupting the class and it had to stop.

It continued on to the point where the student rep came to me and said, "These two are talking all the time and it is affecting my education."

So, I pulled her into my office and we talked, and I could tell she was getting frustrated about something in class. I looked at her and said, "You are exactly the kind of nurse we need. We need leaders, and I know that you are unhappy about this, but I also know that you will do better."

She just came to me and told me that she had been selected as a new grad in the neonatal ICU at Stanford. They have a very prestigious NICU and she's the only new grad who has ever been hired into that unit. She's just awesome.

And to make this story even more poignant, she received our school's Alumni Memorial Award, which is a scholarship that was created in honor of one of our nurse practitioner students. She was a transport nurse and was killed in a helicopter crash. Unbeknownst to anyone at the college, this nurse had just been asked to be the mobile transport nurse for the NICU at Stanford. I don't know what prompted her decision to take this position, but she is certainly an outstanding nurse.

With such high caliber students promoting your nursing program, I would think that nursing schools would have greater recognition in the community.

Nursing education, per se, gets a bad rap from politicians, educators, administrators, even the provosts at many universities as being too expensive. I've actually asked the American Association of Colleges of Nursing (AACN) to write a position paper on what it is like to be an administrator in a nursing program. I have had my job for 11 years, and I have had 4 bosses. By the time you get one up to speed, the next one comes and starts questioning, "Why do you need this many faculty?" Universities have a fair amount of turnover at the top and there hasn't been a great deal written about this issue.

When we talk about our current nursing shortage we have to address things like nursing education, faculty, faculty salaries...

...And how do we make this paradigm shift here. We have a unique situation in California and we have an opportunity to be very futuristic. California ranks 49th in the nation in nurse-to-patient ratios. We have closed BSN programs at the University of California campuses and at USC. While two UC campuses have reinstated nursing programs, we need more BSN and MSN educational programs. Distance educational programs have sprung up, and many people who did get their associate degree have done it in non-traditional ways, so they haven't actually been at a university. Without some time in a university setting, students lose. We have a very under-prepared workforce with very few leaders and role models. We are behind the curve. We are burdened by lack of higher education in nursing, a large geographic state, and a very limited pool to draw from for future faculty.

I think we need to have more BSN- and MSN-prepared nurses in our state. One of the solutions is a program for master's entry level students. I think we should have done these years ago. I am in a health science university, and in every single health profession we offer, the student comes in with a bachelor's degree and continues with his or her professional education. That is what we are currently doing in our nursing program. I have taught at other BSN programs and this is 100% better. You have an academically proven person who has selected nursing as his or her career. They want to be looked at as professionals and are career-focused. BSN programs are great, but we need leaders and faculty. We need a fast track like other professions.

These master's entry students are mature go-getters with great communication skills, critical thinking, and problem solving, and come in with a passionate drive to move up quickly in the profession. The community colleges are still producing the majority of nurses that we need, but we need to develop a more seamless articulation. Morally and professionally, we have a responsibility to elevate the educational level of nursing. Until we do that, we're going to be doing more of the same.

The new paradigm should have 70% that are BSN- and masters-prepared, and 30% community college. Education broadens people's views so you'll have less of that marginalization that occurs in nursing. The arguments comparing and contrasting BSN vs ADN nurses will never go away until we have a higher prepared individual that comes out of the program.

We interviewed a woman for a faculty position and asked for her philosophy of graduate education. She said, "Well, when I was an associate degree nurse, I looked at the world this way. When I was a BSN nurse, I looked at it this way," widening her hands, "then I got my masters and I thought I knew it all. Now I have my PhD and I realize I don't know anything." She continued, "I am a different person."

However, in order to provide more programs, we need more federal money. In Canada, the Ministry of Health outfitted every school of nursing with a simulation center. They understood the schools' need for better equipment. Why don't we do that? Why don't we value nursing to that degree? Why must we place the entire financial burden on the hospitals and schools of nursing? We know it works, so why not do something as broad as that? Why should I spend my time as the dean running after money to get a skills lab together? It should be regional and it should be funded. That would make a big difference.

Simulation is definitely here to stay. We use it beyond clinical training and physical assessment. We use it for scenarios, problem solving, multitasking, and decision making. We've just moved into a larger lab, and our hope is to have 4 simulators that can be programmed so the nursing student can be responsible for 4 patients at a time. These simulators can have pain or be unconscious, and they talk— through the faculty. We are creating a virtual hospital experience.

I think our most immediate goal is to prepare people to be educators, not just flying by the seat of our pants and learning the ropes from an apprentice/mentor model. We need to have people who are educated in curriculum development, evaluation, statistical analysis, and looking at why we do what we do.

We're at a period in time when we need to develop faculty-mentoring models for a whole new breed of faculty. Right now, the majority of faculty are baby-boomers, who work hard and have difficulty finding a balance between work and home life. It's not easy, but I think if you create a healthy culture, it attracts people.

We started the first fully-integrated Web-based curriculum for family nurse practitioners in 1997. We offered a hybrid program of campus-based seminars twice a semester with the curriculum online with discussion boards, etc. This attracted faculty who were innovative, creative, and interested in thinking outside of the box.

We need to take responsibility for educating nurses to be educators. I was very disappointed in the American Association of Critical Care Nurses (AACN) when the Doctor of Nursing Practice (DNP) was in its last iteration. They stated MSN Programs in Education should be phased out and replaced with DNP programs as we need to have expert clinicians teaching in nursing and a MSN in nursing education only prepares a generalist with no added clinical focus. In the first iteration of the DNP curriculums, it was planned that we would be building our educational pool for faculty as well as expert clinicians. The approved DNP Essentials does not provide any educational content to prepare faculty. I am an advocate for DNP Programs and we launched our program in January 2008, but we offer an educational minor. In my opinion we need not only the clinical experts, but also the educational piece to prepare expert faculty.

Every school of nursing should have some way for their faculty to take the core educational classes, whether it's through a Web-based university or a traditional format, but we should demand that.

The National League for Nursing (NLN) is now offering the nurse educator certificate. I don't believe that is enough, but it is a good start. We need to do a better job of educating who is teaching nursing. I think if you looked at other disciplines and you looked at nursing, you'd see that we have a lot of the apprentice model going on as far as teaching. People have not had core instruction in how to write a curriculum or how to evaluate a program.

What should we do in the political arena?

The first thing we should do is look at funding for nursing education. I mentioned the simulation centers, but physician education (years 3 and 4 in their curriculum) is funded by Medicare dollars. I think there should be core funding for all schools of nursing at the university level. The community colleges are already receiving public dollars. I think every school of nursing should receive federal funding. That could be a pipe dream, but when you look at the long-term needs of our society, I believe that is a wise investment. Otherwise, we are going to see more foreign nurses, who are actually depleting nursing in their own countries.

International recruitment is another challenge.

I've been approached by representatives from Indonesia, China, Taiwan, Korea, Philippines, and many other countries about helping them develop nursing programs. They want us to take our intellectual capital and our faculty and educate their schools of nursing on how to develop a BSN program. They've realized that it is an $8 billion industry for the Philippines to export health care professionals. In general, I don't think many deans of nursing find that to be acceptable.

Fifty percent of our nurses who work in California are educated outside of California. They went to school in Wyoming or Montana and they want to move to sunny California. In 2007, the California Board of Registered Nursing (BRN) found, for the very first time, that more nurses are moving out of California than are moving in. We attribute it to the economy, and we are very concerned about that.

So, we are educating only 50% of our nurses to meet California's workforce needs, and now more nurses are moving outside of the state. We're supporting that with outside people and foreign nurses. You can understand why our state has the highest ratio of foreign nurses in the country. That is why I say that in the states that are in dire need, like California, we have to have base funding in schools of nursing.

We need enough resources in order to add faculty, not recruit nurses from foreign countries. We think there were between 14,000 and 19,000 students who were turned away from schools of nursing in California in the last 2 years. That might not be a completely accurate number because people apply to multiple schools, but it shows that there is enough interest in our own state to satisfy our nursing needs. We don't even need nurses educated outside of California. We just need to be able to educate the ones that we have in our own state. The problem is we don't have enough schools of nursing.

We need to make DNP programs and PhD programs affordable. We need to provide financial incentives for people to move on to become educators. We can't have more nurses without more educators.

I think there needs to be parity in faculty salaries. We've looked at the workforce model where you pay more for professions at risk. For example, in some universities if you have an MBA program, their faculty is paid more than those in geography. Right now, nursing faculty starting as assistant professors, in most situations, make less than a new ADN nurse in our state. We have to elevate faculty salaries.

We need to have more leadership development so that we can communicate at the table. In the leadership class that I'm teaching for the DNP program, I'm having the students read a book on facilitation and how to run a meeting. That is a core skill that everybody needs to have before they graduate. We are the team coordinators. Everybody should be able to be an expert facilitator and speaker. Unfortunately, I think nursing has always explained things in a circular fashion. We need to communicate clearly and concisely. We must be better at articulating our profession, our roles, and what we contribute as team members. I think communication is a huge area.

The BSN should be completely reevaluated. I am pleased with the new BSN Essentials (AACN 2008, The Essentials of Baccalaureate Education for Professional Nursing Practice, October 20, 2008); however, one of my thoughts over the years to advance the profession in our state would be for everyone to go to the community college for their associate degree and the 5 content areas in nursing, then transfer to a university to complete their RN, BSN (take the NCLEX), and then graduate with a master's degree in nursing. That's probably not going to happen, but we need to make some fundamental changes to create more master's prepared nurses.

How would you respond to the arguments that you are limiting entry into practice to only those who can afford a baccalaureate degree or higher?

Well, we just have to get over that. We have to do what is best for the patients. We have to do what is best for the profession. And we have to do what is best for society. If you just keep focused on those 3 things, then you are going in the right direction. Do we ask our Physician Assistants (PAs) if they would prefer to go to a community college first and get their certificate, because it is too expensive to get a master's degree? We don't have those dialogues.

This is a paradigm shift, and we need to do what is right for the profession.

What are your proudest accomplishments to date?

I actually have 3.

The first is starting the Master's of Science in Nursing Entry (MSN-E) program where you take the 4-year individuals and put them through an accelerated BSN curriculum, then they continue on to get a master's degree. Those nurses are, in my opinion, the best nurses we have in Southern California right now. I'm not saying that we are the best of the best, but we select the right students. We interview all of our candidates from a very large pool and make sure they are a good fit for nursing. That has worked very well for us. We are very excited. We get nothing but rave reviews from our clinical partners.

Secondly, I'm very proud of the integration of simulation as an active learning tool.

Finally, I am excited to be teaching in the DNP program. It is very rewarding to teach this caliber of student. After working with these students, reading their papers, and following their critical thinking, I'm very excited about the future. There is hope after I retire. You've got people who want to change the health care system. They're creative and energetic and enthusiastic.

There are more DNP programs popping up in the United States, which makes sense. What does the PhD nursing educator do for clinical practice? Not very much. They are expert researchers, but lose their clinical focus. We need PhD-prepared nurses, please do not misunderstand me; but, at a time when we have a severe faculty shortage, we need to assure all DNP-prepared nurses are expert educators as well. I believe the DNP graduate will make a big difference for us, and provide a big intellectual elevation in clinical nursing.

Do you consider your work to be heroic?

I do. I think one of the reasons is that being a dean at a school of nursing is incredibly hard work and complex. My forte is administration. I think I have a good knack for getting the right people on the bus, of being open-minded and visionary. I think I am also very good at empowering faculty to be who they want to be in their growth. I don't think we have a lot of leaders like that in schools of nursing. I'm more fortunate because I'm at a private university. I don't have as much bureaucracy to deal with as do other places.

I think where I've been heroic is I've achieved high levels of accreditation for our college with limited resources. I've fought administrative battles to obtain recognition as an undervalued profession at our university. Private universities do not receive public funding so we have to work harder. I also remain very excited about the profession and I think I communicate that.

I have incredible satisfaction from all of my years in nursing. I wouldn't trade it for anything. We have all had those special experiences. I had one when I was the evening supervisor working in the ICU.

This gentleman had suffered a severe heart attack and had a high prognosis for dying. His physician was treating him very conservatively, and instead of giving Lasix IV, his doctor prescribed it orally. He was in heart failure and just limping along. I just treated him respectfully and took the lead from his wife and had a pleasant experience. Eventually he was moved out of the unit because he no longer warranted the ICU care and his doctor wasn't really treating him.

About 8 years later, I was shopping in the grocery store and this woman was chasing me down the aisle saying, "There you are. There you are." I didn't know what to think and wanted to avoid her. She finally came up to me and said, "I have been looking for you for 8 years to thank you for taking care of my husband. You are the only nurse who gave me hope that my husband would survive. I wanted to tell you that we have had 8 wonderful years. We bought a travel trailer and we have done so much! Thank you so much for what you did for me and my husband."

What a wonderful experience, and a lovely story.

It was unbelievable. So whenever I have a bad day, I think of those experiences. There have been so many good things along the way.

Karen Hanford, EdD (c), MSN, FNP
Founding Dean, College of Graduate Nursing
California

CHAPTER 7

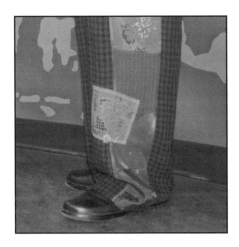

The Value of a Nurse

I always wanted to be an actress. It was my girlfriend who wanted to be a nurse. She convinced me to come with her to be a candy striper and, as it turned out, she became the actress, and I became the nurse!

I have been a nurse for nearly 40 years, and pediatrics has always been my specialty. I remember my first job in pediatrics. I loved it so much that I thought that they didn't even have to pay me.

Do you remember your salary when you first started?

Absolutely. I was paid $365 per month! That was when we were taught that nurses are loyal, nurses are selfless, nurses don't strike— even if it meant that they couldn't support their families on their salaries. However, in the 1970s when everything was up for grabs, so was nursing. We started to take a stand for ourselves as real people—not just servants.

Nursing changed. And I'm glad that it did.

Where has your career taken you?

I continued to gain more experience and education in pediatric nursing. I also pursued nursing education and staff development. Education rejuvenates me. I love nursing and always strive to promote nurses, regardless of location.

I recently returned from a medical mission trip to Sucre, Bolivia sponsored by the Joliet (Illinois) diocese. They have a hospital there and needed an educator to instruct the nurses. My interpreter told me that I should begin by teaching them specific skills, but I wanted to assess the situation first. The nurses were very resistant and told me, "We don't want you to just come in here and criticize us and tell us we're doing things the wrong way." My response was that it was never my intention to do that. I'm a staff developer. I promote and increase knowledge. I try to help nurses find their own potential, their own strength, and their own power.

Once they realized that I was there to enhance their own skills, I was accepted. I found that while the nurses in Bolivia had good technical skills, they didn't have very good self-esteem. I tried to provide them with more dignity as nurses.

What is your message to nurses here and abroad?

Nursing is a very honorable profession, and we do so much more than we realize.

Francine Gust, MS, RN, C
Nurse Educator
Illinois

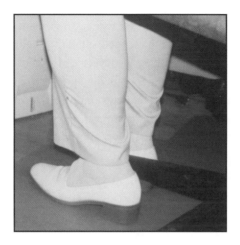

CHAPTER 8

Not Just a Piece of Paper

I am named after my great-grandmother, who was a midwife in a small town in Texas. I didn't know about her practice until a few years ago when I was working on getting my certification to be a lactation consultant. My grandmother proudly told me, "That is what your great-grandmother did! The one you are named after."

There isn't a better profession to go into; the opportunities are limitless. Both of my sisters work in health care, and my daughters are nurses as well. My older daughter is a nurse on an organ transplant unit, and my younger daughter is in nursing school. It's in our genes!

My background is in pediatric nursing, and I was a very aggressive peds ICU nurse. My personality serves me well in my current role as a case manager for the hospital. I will do whatever it takes to make sure my patients receive the appropriate care in the fastest time possible.

Can you share a story that explains how you work?

The other day a gentleman showed up at my office. In very broken

English, he said, "I have a problem with the doctor, and they told me you would fix it."

His wife had been seen by their regular physician, and he thought she had cancer. They called the specialist but they couldn't be seen for at least 6 weeks. Of course, they were very concerned.

I got the information and called the specialist, and was able to make an appointment for 9 AM the next morning. I will not work with a physician who doesn't put his patients first.

My work as a case manager is very important. I never lose sight of the fact that there is a real person behind every piece of paper and patient file I'm working on.

Virginia Wilhelm, RN
Case Manager
Illinois

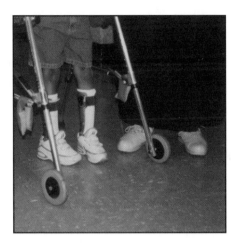

CHAPTER 9

Magnificent Little Steps

O ne of the differences between hospital nursing and community (school) nursing is that you can really create your own role here. I tell nurses who ask me about school nursing that it's up to them to make it a challenge.

How long have you been a nurse?

It's been 36 years! I started in adult rehabilitation for a year, then left to raise my family. When my children were in kindergarten, I discovered that the school had nurses and they immediately began encouraging me to volunteer. They were promoting their profession in such a positive way that they hooked me! It was the gentle guidance of those nurses that encouraged me to do the work I am doing today.

Can you give a brief overview of school nurses?

We have a tiered system of nurses. Illinois requires that school nurses have a state certification, which is a Type 73 certificate. We also have program nurses, and 1:1 classroom nurses. There are multiple nurses in the school, but their roles are all slightly different.

We do a lot of anticipation and prevention. In regular education, we would be working directly with the child, but in the special needs setting we help guide the team. As our children here become more medically complex our program nurse has been able to blend nursing into the classroom.

In the chronic care setting you are thrilled when even the smallest gains are made, and those first steps are taken. We really look for those magnificent little steps that make a difference, even though it may take years.

Looking over the course of your career, what has given you the greatest sense of accomplishment?

There are so many things. In the early part of my career, I gained the most satisfaction from making inroads to getting appropriate medical care for the children. In years past, I remember when doctors would come out to the car to examine a special needs child because they didn't want them in their office. I was able to locate the right doctors and connect them with these families. Being an advocate for a parent is getting the best medical attention for their child. I feel really good about that role.

Do you consider your work heroic?

I see myself as a teacher, a mentor and definitely an advocate for children with special needs, but I don't think I'm a hero.

Judy Gray, RN, MS
Pediatric Nurse Practitioner/School Nurse Practitioner
Illinois

CHAPTER 10

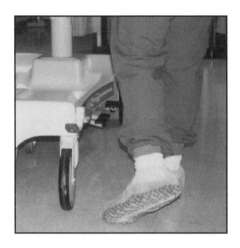

In Step With the Future

I've been a nurse for more than 25 years! I have worked in critical care and telemetry, but I really found my niche in surgery. I like working with my hands, and with my First Assistant (FA) designation, I am able to make and suture incisions under the surgeon's supervision.

I love anatomy and I have a strong desire to learn. Surgery is fascinating to me because I can learn about, and participate in, a variety of areas. You can specialize in ophthalmic cases, or orthopedics, neurology, urology, cardiology, gynecology or plastic surgery, among others. Of course, there's always general surgery.

The other day one of the surgeons asked me to suture his patient and he laughed and said, "I'll make a surgeon out of you yet!"

"Oh no you won't," I replied. "I have no desire to be a surgeon. I'm very happy being a nurse."

Would you recommend nursing as a career option for your sons?

Of course. I think that there are tremendous career opportunities in nursing, especially for men. I love what I do. Most importantly I hope that my children see that, because there is nothing worse than being in a profession that you don't like.

Would you consider anything that you've done in your nursing practice to be heroic?

I think that it's heroic to even have the love that I have for my profession. I'm lucky. I still love what I do, but the nursing shortage is making it difficult for us. People don't consider nursing to be a career option anymore, so there is more work to do and fewer people to do it.

Any final thoughts....

I'd like to share the following quote from Florence Nightingale:

No system can endure that does not march.
Are we walking to the future or to the past?
Are we progressing or are we stereotyping?
We remember that we have scarcely crossed the threshold
of uncivilized civilization in Nursing;
there is still so much to do.
Don't let us stereotype mediocrity.
We are still on the threshold of Nursing.

Kim Opalacz, RN, BS, FA
Clinical Nurse Manager
Illinois

CHAPTER 11

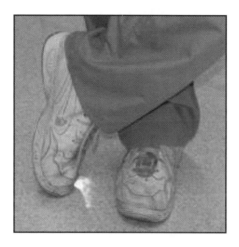

Like Father....

Being a nurse runs in families, and I've tried to capture that in a few of the stories in this book. We usually picture a daughter who's following in her mother's footsteps, but with the next 2 stories we'll learn how a father and his son share more than the typical parent-child relationship...

I'm so glad you asked me if I had any combat boots in my nursing shoes collection, because I hadn't interviewed any military nurses up to this point.

My son, Sam, is a nurse in the Army and he's currently stationed in Baghdad. I thought you might be interested in talking to him because of everything that's been going on since 9/11, and get the soldier's perspective.

I would love to talk with him. This book is a snapshot of America's nurses today, and right now we are

providing nursing and medical attention to our troops involved in conflicts overseas. I welcome the opportunity to speak with him, but it's really interesting to me that you're a nurse too. Were you in the military as well?

I am a retired Army Major, but I started out in the Air Force. My father retired from the Air Force, and when I was in the seventh grade, he suffered a heart attack. They took him to the Navy hospital close to home, and I don't know if the person taking care of him was a corpsman or a nurse, but my father spoke so highly of him and all that he had done for him that I think that's what put the spark in my head. I decided to join the Air Force and was guaranteed a job working in a hospital.

After basic training and tech school my first assignment was in labor and delivery, and the newborn nursery. I never expected that assignment but as an Air Force medic, I ended up being more involved in the room setup and cleanup than actually taking care of patients. One thing I did learn there, however, was how to start an IV. I don't know how it's done on the civilian side but in the military it's, "watch one, do one, teach one" and that's literally how it went.

From there I went to ICU and then to the ER. I left the Air Force and joined the Reserves while I was going to nursing school and after graduation I came back to the military, but this time in the Army. The Army offered me a better career path than the Air Force did. They guaranteed an assignment for me and the potential for promotion. I eventually went back to grad school and became an acute care nurse practitioner. I'm now a retired Army Major, working as a critical care nurse in a military hospital.

Why did you choose the ICU?

I felt that I could make a difference there. I've always liked the ICU and ER, and I think it's for the same reason that Sam does. It's the adrenaline; the rush of not knowing what to expect.

When did Sam become interested in your work?

He has always been the kind of person who likes to be in the middle of everything, right in the center of the action, so it didn't surprise me at all that he would be interested in the ER. He's always been a high energy kind of guy, and has always been interested in what I was doing.

One of my assignments was at the burn unit in San Antonio, and I was asked to develop classes for the Air Force flight team on how to take care of burn patients. I was preparing slides of my patients and my son wanted me to do the lecture for his class at school. I told him, "You know Sam, I'm not sure the kids really want to see this gruesome stuff." He was only in the third grade at the time.

We had a bring-your-kids-to-work day, when I was stationed in Germany. I took all 3 of my children, but one of the sergeants asked Sam if he wanted to start an IV and he replied, "Sure," as if it was the most natural thing in the world. I don't know why this guy would let a 10-year-old child stick him, but Sam really enjoyed that.

I think that was the start of his interest in nursing and the military. He wanted to do that for a living, so I told him, "If that's what you want to do, I'll support you on it," and that's what I did.

He's a great kid. His brother and sister kid him all the time because he'll say things and they'll say, "You sound just like Dad." We also look alike, and what's even more interesting is that we're born on the same day. So I guess it doesn't surprise me that he chose the career he did.

Can you tell me about your work in the burn unit? That's also a very specialized place to practice.

I would have to say that of all my assignments, the burn unit was my most challenging and most interesting experience. The Army had a burn flight team that would fly, literally, all over the world and transport patients back to our unit. There was a German Air Force base accident that happened back in 1988 and I was stateside, prepping for the patients who were burned in that airplane collision. I also remember a

43

helicopter crash in Korea where we sent over a team to bring back 13 patients. We would admit both military and civilian patients from all over the world, because ours was such a well-known research facility.

Would you mind telling me a little about your patients in the burn unit?

All of our patients suffered significant burns. The first patient I ever had came back a year or two after he was discharged, and asked if I knew who he was. I had no idea, but when he told me his name I immediately remembered his story. He was only 26 years old, and was a passenger in a dune buggy. His friend was driving down a trail, lost control of the vehicle and hit a tree. The gas tank which is located in the front, exploded, causing flames to engulf the front seat. He sustained extremely severe burns. I remember taking care of him. He had so many surgeries, debridements, and grafts all over his body. We'd also have to treat the donor sites like other burns. It was a long, slow healing process.

We would also see children, which was always tough. I remember one little boy who had burns to his upper extremity, face, and head. The occupational therapist measured him for his Jobst stockings (compression garments), that he'd have to wear over the burned areas. It was Halloween, so they decided to get him the black Jobst and put a Batman emblem on his head. It turned out great for him—he loved it!

It was a very collaborative environment. We also had a residency program. Physicians would graduate in July and would be expected to make decisions on their own. It was interesting because you would find that after about 6 months they would start asking questions again. They were learning on their own, but before making a final decision, they would look your way for reassurance.

I was lucky enough to work under 2 leading edge physicians who were specialists in the field of burn care and research. The Commander was the man in charge. He was brilliant, but he could also be mean. I was there for 6 months before he even grunted at me as we passed in the hallway. I knew I had arrived though, because he normally wouldn't even look in your direction.

I remember an incident when I was working the night shift and had to give a report to an Air Force surgeon. He was doing his 30-day surgical rotation on our unit and wasn't familiar with our protocols. I finished my report and made a suggestion about what to do next for the patient, but he dismissed me, saying, "Oh no, we're doing this instead." I told him that what he ordered wasn't what was normally done, to which he replied, "I'm the doctor and this is what we're going to do." The following morning, instead of going home we all decided to stay for morning rounds with the Commander. When he read through the patient's chart he demanded to know who wrote the orders. We just looked at the surgeon and our doctor looked at us and asked, "Why didn't you tell him our protocol?" "Sir," we started, "we tried to tell him what to do last night." So he turned to this young physician and said, "The next time my nurses tell you to do something, you do it."

We had our satisfaction, and left shortly afterward. The Commander knew that we knew more than the physicians did and supported us, but he was still a mean guy. (laugh)

How were you able to replenish yourself when you worked with this patient population?

When I look back I realize that I never socialized with any of the people I worked with. When I left work, I left it behind and went home to my wife and 3 children. My family was probably my saving grace at that point. At home I was involved in sports and Scouts and school, and I learned to separate my work from my family life. I hate to sound callous but I couldn't let myself become involved with the patients or their families.

What types of patients do you most enjoy working with? What type of work gives you the most satisfaction?

I enjoy working with the sickest patients in the unit because they are the ones who will challenge me the most. That's why I like working in the ICU. I feel that I make a difference. The patient will never know what I did, and that's okay because I know what I did. The family might not even know everything that I did for their loved one, but I know that at the end of the day, I can walk away from the unit knowing I did a good job. This person is better now than when I showed up in the morning. That is what gives me satisfaction.

Have you ever considered your work to be heroic?

Not really. I've never considered myself a hero of any kind. I'm not out on the front lines fighting the bad guys. I think I do my job, and I do it well, but I've never considered myself a hero.

Have you ever been involved in a conflict overseas?

You know, I never was. I was in the military during the invasion of Granada and Panama, and I was on the burn unit for the first Gulf War, but that lasted such a short time. We were gearing up to expand our unit from 15 beds to 150 beds, but there were no patients, which was good. And then I retired just before the push for Iraq, so I missed it all.

On the other hand Sam is right there in Baghdad, and as much as I'd like to think this won't affect him, this is going to change him forever. It's a double-edged sword. I'm proud that he's there and that he's doing this for his country, but on the other side of the coin, he's my son and I'd hate to see anything happen to him. They grow up so quickly, faster than they do here in the States. What he has seen and what he has had to do, I hope he never has to see and do again. I really hope that.

Chad Matta, RN, CCRN
Major, US Army, Retired
Critical Care Nurse
Georgia

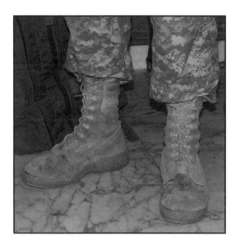

CHAPTER 12

....Like Son

I really appreciate the fact that you're calling me from work for this interview. I should mention that "work" is the 86th Combat Support Hospital inside Baghdad's "green zone" in Iraq.

Not a problem. I apologize for not being able to talk earlier. We didn't have anything going on all day and then 10 minutes before our appointment we got a radio call that there were 7 patients inbound. I work in the ER and one of my patients came in because of an explosion that pushed a wall on top of him. It broke his ribs and pelvis, and punctured both lungs. He came in cool, clammy, diaphoretic, breathing 45 times a minute, and in severe pain. I gave him pain medication; we intubated him, inserted bilateral chest tubes, stabilized his pelvis, and sent him to the OR.

While he was in our unit, I could see his heart rate and respiratory rate come down and see his blood pressure improve. I felt like I fixed a problem and provided him with some relief from that pain. It's a great feeling when you can insert a 12-gauge needle in your patient's chest and see that whoosh of air come out, and know that you're making a difference.

It's a very fast-paced, high-adrenaline environment that I just thrive on. I love being in this environment, and I love providing care to the soldiers who are out there risking their lives on a daily basis. To me, this is the ultimate career experience.

You sound so passionate about your work. Have you always been interested in nursing as a career?

I've always been interested in the medical profession. My dad is a nurse. He retired from the Army as a Nurse Corps officer, although he started out as a medic for the Air Force. He's a critical care nurse, and we moved all over the world with him. He worked in the burn unit at the Army Institute of Surgical Research in Texas, which is where we send our burn patients. He was on the flight team there, which plays into my life today. From there we moved to Germany where he worked at Landstuhl Military Hospital. That's where we evacuate our soldiers, before they head back home to the United States.

So, I've always been around military hospitals and, because of my dad's connections, I've had great opportunities to shadow nurses and medics at work. I've had some great experiences. I started my first IV when I was 10 years old. It was bring-your-child-to-work day and he took me, and my brother and sister, to the clinic where he was the chief nurse. It was great because he taught us how to do splints, and took us to the lab where we spun down blood and learned how to do urine dip sticks. That's where I started the IV on the medic. We all wanted to do it, but I won because I was the oldest.

If you look at the 3 of us today, you'll see that we're all in health care. My brother is in a post-graduate physical therapy program, and my sister is a massage therapist and is enrolled in a nursing program. And to round it all out, my mom is an occupational therapist.

Growing up, I was a physical therapy assistant and a Red Cross Volunteer, and I learned a lot from my dad. I just ate it up; it was my favorite thing. If you were to see a picture of us, you'd see that my dad and I look a lot alike. Some of my best friends actually call us twins, which is kind of fitting because we even have the same personality. The scariest part is (laughing...) we were born on the same day! I was his birthday present when he turned 25.

So, following in your father's footsteps and becoming an Army nurse was practically a foregone conclusion.

In fact, there are 3 people in my senior command at this hospital who worked with him, and everyone at the hospital knows him. Every time I run into someone who worked with him, I apologize for anything he ever did to them (laughing)...just kidding. I like my dad and he was good at what he did, so I've never run into anyone who's held a grudge against him.

Were you nervous at all about being deployed to Iraq?

I volunteered to come over here. I am here because there are guys out there doing things that are far more dangerous. I am working in what is essentially a stateside facility, with a higher acuity.

We are a 10-bed emergency room, which seems small compared to the hospital I came from in the States. We also see a much different patient population. The medical problem has to be either life threatening, threatening to a limb, or to eyesight.

The Chief of the ER once said, "In this environment, the violence of action is more important than intelligence of thought sometimes." Which means do something, whether it's starting an IV, administering oxygen, or placing a patient on a monitor. If you're going to do something, do it hard, do it fast, and do it smoothly. There's also a fine line between being quick and efficient and freaking out. And then go on and do something else. Don't keep focused on the small, minute things; there's a bigger picture to everything.

Most of the guys we treat are very, very happy that we are here. We'll get them off the aircraft or one of their buddies will bring them in, and once they're here they feel like they're at home base. They believe that if they can just make it to the Cash, then their buddy's going to be okay. For my part, I love that I'm able to provide care to a patient population that is grateful that we're there. They deserve all the care that I'm going to give them.

When you say, "make it to the Cash" what exactly do you mean?

That's how we refer to our hospital: the Combat Support House, or CSH. We just call it "Cash".

I'm guessing that you might experience a culture shock when you come back here and work in the ER. When you describe soldiers bringing in their buddies and being grateful for your help, I couldn't help but be reminded of an experience a friend of mine had when she was working in the emergency department of a trauma center in Chicago. A car screeched to a stop at the emergency entrance, and the bloodied body of a gunshot victim was pushed out of the back seat. The driver honked his horn for attention, and then sped off.

I've already experienced that. Two out of the 3 emergency thoracotomies we did in the ER back home were on patients who were kicked out on our front door. Same situation as yours. It's really a different environment back home.

What is the best thing about working at the CSH?

I love the staff here. That's probably the best thing I can say. It's an all military staff, and it's all people who want to be here. We have a very tight knit family. That's what concerns me about coming back to the States. There will always be those few people who don't get along with everybody else, or who don't work as a team. We haven't run into that here.

Everyone here knows that this environment is artificial though, and that we'll probably never run into this again in our careers. We all talk about it, so we're very aware of what to expect when we go home.

You've been in Iraq for nearly a year, and have seen firsthand the injuries and trauma our soldiers are sustaining. What do you think we need to do to prepare for our men and women who will be seeking medical attention back home at the VA?

I honestly think we're going to see a lot of mild traumatic brain injury (MTBI) diagnoses. These patients will be experiencing memory loss and unexplained behavioral and cognitive issues. I think we'll also see more post traumatic stress disorder (PTSD) diagnoses. These patients might not need hospitalization, but they'll need support on an outpatient basis.

We've seen a significant amount of amputees in this conflict as well. We're getting so good at wearing our body armor that we don't see as many thoracic and abdominal injuries. Extremities are very vulnerable in this environment.

One small piece of equipment has saved so many lives here, and that is the tourniquet. I've seen guys live with bilateral lower extremity amputations because their buddy put tourniquets on both their legs and stopped the bleeding. It's amazing. Every single soldier who comes into this theater is given several tourniquets, and I believe that has saved lives.

What are your career plans for the next 5 years?

I'll probably be out of the military. My dream job, and this goes back to my dad, is doing life flight critical care transport. My dream job is actually in Austin, Texas, and it's a program called Star Life Flight. It's a multi-mission helicopter EMS program that does critical care transport throughout the hospitals in the area. They do scene flight, where they fly to the scene of an accident and pick up a patient. They also do search and rescue, both on the ground and in the water. They fly for the fire department doing fire suppression, and for the local police. That's my ultimate goal.

What does your father think of your career?

I think my dad is unbelievably proud of me. He really loves what I'm doing. He came to see me off when I left Ft. Campbell, and just before we left he said, "Half of me wants to go with you and the other half thinks you're out of your mind." I know he doesn't want me to be in a dangerous situation, but I believe I'm in far less danger than the guys doing the real Army job. I'm there to make sure they get the highest level of care if they get injured. I've always been that way, and my mom tells me that my dad was the exact same way when he was my age.

You've found your niche.

Yeah. I love it, I really do.

Would you consider your actions to be heroic?

No. Not a single one of them. I mean, other people might think so, but I think that for an action to be considered heroic, you shouldn't enjoy doing it. I'm not doing anything I don't want to do. I love doing my job. Don't tell anybody else, but I would do this job for no money, I like it that much. My goal in life is to wake up every morning and actually want to go to work.

Sam Matta, RN, CEN
EMT Nurse
Captain, Army Nurse Corps
Currently deployed to Iraq with 86th CSH

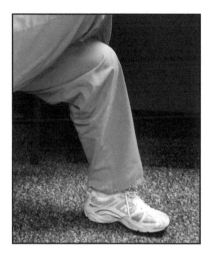

CHAPTER 13

Patient-Centered Care

Is there any other kind of care?

Sadly, there are many places where the patient is never even considered. We don't accept that here. Even though it might seem obvious, we need to tell everyone that we provide patient-centered care.

My mother is a very smart woman and she's been in health care her whole life. I was having trouble with something one day and she said, "As a nurse, making decisions is very easy. You simply ask yourself, 'Is this the right thing for the patient?' If the answer is no, you do everything in your power not to let that happen. If the answer is yes, you do everything in your power to make it happen. If it's right for the patient, then it will be right for the nurses, and the nurses will be happy. Their performance will be better, which will make the institution happy, which will make the Board happy." It really is that simple.

We recently admitted a 41-year-old patient to the ICU with shortness of breath and a broken leg. Apparently, she fell while trying to go to the bathroom. Her breathing was so bad we eventually had to intubate her and put her on a ventilator. In the meantime, she had to have surgery to repair the fracture. Did I mention she weighed 450 pounds? The surgery could have been done as an outpatient procedure if it weren't for the complications from her weight, which also affected her breathing.

After some time on the unit, I got the nurses together to talk about our plan for this patient. We had a morbidly obese patient who was non-weight bearing for the next 3 months, and who was on a ventilator. To make matters worse, we didn't have the right equipment to manage her weight. Well, we found a company on the Internet that carried the right equipment: bed, chair, and lift, but it would be a week before they could send it. "Forget it," I told the company rep, "she'll be dead in a week." That was a little extreme, I know, but the company called me back and said the equipment was on its way.

When the furniture arrived, a few of the nurses and I went to her room and told her that we had a new bed and chair for her. She looked at us and mouthed the word "why?" I was confused. I told her that we got her a new bed so she'd be more comfortable, and that we had ordered other things to help her get out of bed and into a chair. Again, she asked why. I couldn't understand this. Why wasn't she happy about changing her bed and being more comfortable?

"Do you like this one?" I asked. "Does it help you move around in bed?"

She mouthed the words, "A new bed is fine, but why are you bothering?"

I needed to understand what this patient was thinking, so I got down close to her and said, "Jenny, what's the problem here? Why don't you want to move? Are you afraid of something? We're just trying to help you."

I'll never forget her response: "Why do you care?"

That just hit me. I explained, "We care because you're our patient and we've grown to like you, and we hope you've grown to like us."

"But I'm so fat," she mouthed, as she looked away.

I said, "You used to be fat but now you've lost 80 pounds. You used to smoke 2 packs of cigarettes a day, and now you don't. It's as if you've gone to one of those places in California or Arizona where people go to lose a lot of weight. Think of it that way and now it's time to have fun!"

"But no one's ever cared," she said at last.

I told her that she finally met a group that does.

So now she gets up with minimal assistance and scoots herself along in a wheelchair, and is planning on going home. And it's all because somebody took the time to look at her as a person and not as a daunting challenge.

But it is a challenge in a critical care setting.

Actually, the patients in an ICU and the patients on a general medical/surgical unit are basically the same. It's the equipment that's different. When you get down to it they all need a bath and they still need to eat. They need the same care and attention, so don't get carried away with the machines. Move them out of your way.

I didn't go into nursing just to do what I was told. I want to sit and talk to people, get to know them, and have them get to know me. I like it when a patient asks me about my family. I think we need to share our stories; make people laugh and cry. Our patients just want 5 minutes of our time.

Can you share another instance of true patient-centered care?

I remember getting a call from the admitting department to help a patient out of his van and get a chest x-ray. I don't know why they called me, maybe I was first on their rolodex or something, but I said I'd be there right away. I knew I'd need help, so I called the manager of the cardiac cath lab to help me. He never questioned me. The only thing he asked was, "Can I take the elevator or should I run down the stairs?" I said, "Run down the stairs."

Three years ago, that would have been a fiasco at this hospital. Today, the philosophy at Bert Fish Memorial Hospital is, "The patient needs it. Let's just do it."

When I met the manager at the patient's van, I told him that the 2 of us would have to transfer the gentleman out of his van and into a wheelchair. Then we'd have to transport him to Radiology for a chest x-ray. We assessed the situation and realized the gentleman had dementia, probably Alzheimer's, and was laughing at everything we did. We finally got him into the wheelchair, and by this time all 3 of us were laughing!

We thought we were in the home stretch when we arrived in Radiology, but the patient wouldn't submit to an x-ray unless we went with him. So, we both put on the heavy lead aprons and supported the patient on either side for his chest x-ray. They shot the x-ray but there was too much movement and the image was blurred, so I told the gentleman to be still for the next shot. The technician heard this and said, "He's not the one who's moving. It's the two of you, laughing! Can you both be still?"

It wasn't our job, specifically, to help this patient get his chest x-ray, but the patient needed help and we just did it. I'm glad we did because we learned later that he had several broken ribs.

Over the course of your career, is there a story that stands out for you? An encounter with a patient that has somehow stayed with you?

Probably the most amazing experience I've had with a patient happened early on in my career. I'm certain it won't mean much to anyone else, but it made a lasting impression on me.

Many years ago, I was working the afternoon shift on a unit that had 48 patients. We were staffed with 2 RNs, an LPN and a nurse's aide. It was busy! One of my patients was a nun who came in with abdominal pain and ended up having stomach cancer. It was bad, and had metastasized. I was so drawn to her, like you can be with some patients. Her name was Sara.

One day I was passing her room, and it was right in the middle of my busiest time with patient care and passing medications. She called out from her room, "Kelly, come and sit down for a minute."

I said, "All right, but I don't have much time."

"How long have you been a nurse?"

I told her, and I asked if I could ask her a question.

"Anything," she answered.

"Why did you choose this? Why a nun?" We had a good relationship by this time and I felt comfortable asking her this question. There was something about Sara that was inexplicably fascinating to me.

She told me that it was a calling, and she knew from a very young age that this was what she was going to do. "It's a similar reason to why you're a nurse, isn't it?"

That struck me, and I told her she was right. "But didn't you want to get married and have children?" I asked her.

"Don't you want more staff? Isn't there another way that you'd like to get your work done?" she asked back.

That made me realize we had more in common than I thought. She stayed on our unit for a while and we continued having our conversations and one day I just had to know how she was coping with her diagnosis.

"Sara," I asked, "aren't you angry about having cancer? Don't you want to ask, 'Why? Why me, Lord?' You've followed the Lord all your life and now you've got cancer. Aren't you mad?"

And she said, "No, I have faith that it's going to be okay."

I felt that I was angrier than she was and wanted her to know that I thought it was unfair that she got the short end of the stick.

But she corrected me, "No, I got the long end of the stick. This was meant to be and it'll be okay because I have faith, don't you?"

I told her I didn't think so. She was on chemotherapy and her hair was falling out and I couldn't believe that things were going to be okay for her. That's when she turned the conversation to me. "Kelly? Do you think nursing was the right choice for you?"

I said, "Absolutely, but we're not talking about me."

And she said, "Well, I want to talk about you. Do you think you can make a difference?"

"Of course I can," I responded.

"Well, I've made a difference, too. I think I've made a difference in your life. I think you'll remember me for a long time."

I said I certainly would! I told her that she'd remember me for a long time as well, and we both laughed.

Unfortunately, Sara died the next day.

About 2 months later I received a card from her sister, telling me how much I meant to Sara. She had asked her sister to send me a card after she died to remind me that I made the right choice in becoming a nurse, and that I will make a difference.

I believe she was put there, on my unit, for a reason. At the time I was taking care of 24 patients and felt like no one cared that we were working our fingers to the bone—but it was the right thing to do. I don't know where she came from and I have often wondered if she even existed, but she was meant to be in that room.

All these people, there is a reason why they're here. Stop the madness, sit down and talk with them. That's all they want, just 5 minutes of your time. Take the gloves off your hands and touch them. I always tell nurses not to walk away from a patient without touching him. I guarantee he'll want to grab your hand and not let go.

Kelly Hansen, RN, BSN
Nurse Manager, ICU/PCU
Florida

SECTION TWO

"Wherever men have lived there is a story to be told."

Henry David Thoreau

CHAPTER 14

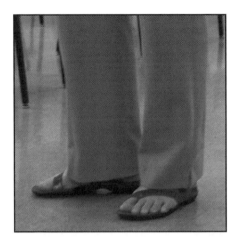

An Open Window

I have had a very eclectic career. I wouldn't call it a traditional nursing career, but I think everything I have done has been enhanced because of my nursing background.

When I first graduated, I worked in intensive care at a very prominent teaching hospital in Chicago. This was in the 1980s and we were experiencing one of our cyclical nursing shortages. I was exploring career opportunities and was interested in leadership and administration. Interestingly enough, when I sat down with my nurse managers and asked for career advice, they told me that there was no reason to get a master's degree in nursing unless I wanted to become a Clinical Nurse Specialist. They told me that I should pursue an MBA instead.

No one was pushing for nursing at that time, which might be part of the reason for today's nursing faculty shortage. We had no succession planning as a profession. We didn't have a clear understanding of how to perpetuate our profession and we weren't setting ourselves up for the next generation of nursing faculty.

I wasn't interested in a clinical program, and the MBA didn't seem like the right fit so I chose the middle of the road, which was a Public Administration/Public Service degree with a focus in Health Care. What I got out of that experience was just how much misunderstanding there is of nursing. It amazes me that unless you could describe yourself in a clinical position, such as a nurse midwife or nurse anesthetist, you were looked at differently. There wasn't a lot of validation for nursing leadership at that time unless you chose a more clinical route. I was interested in the nursing shortage and wanted to know why people weren't choosing nursing as a career.

I had a theory. I had heard all of the other theories about low wages, having to work a variety of shifts, weekends and holidays, having to deal with authority, and even having to work with extreme trauma and illness, but I wanted to explore another avenue. My graduate classes were comprised of a variety of professionals from the public service sector, and included several police officers. It struck me that our professions shared quite a few similarities. We worked the same hours and had to be available 24/7. Their pay was similar, if not less than ours. They also saw the worst of society, but from a criminal perspective, and were exposed to very emotional issues. But police officers weren't experiencing a shortage of recruits.

One difference I identified was that police officers were paid a salary and nurses were paid an hourly wage. The literature says that professionals are paid a salary and hourly workers are in a different category. So for my master's thesis I surveyed all of the hospitals in Chicago and took a look at how they paid nurses. I had a huge response but never really got an answer to my question.

That was an interesting question, though. In my first nursing position I was paid a salary and never punched a clock. I worked in a very progressive hospital and Dr. Luther Christman was the chief nurse. I thought that was how all hospitals operated. Later, at another hospital, I remember thinking that it didn't seem very professional to be talking about paying charge nurses 25 cents more per hour, or whatever the going rate was.

That's right. And now let's take a look at how nursing is portrayed in the media. At the time I was in school there were several police dramas on television, from *Miami Vice* to *Hill Street Blues*. At the same time there was a program about nurses called *Nightingales*. Any nurse who saw that program had to laugh—or be insulted, and enough were insulted that there was a public outcry and the program was cancelled. I don't believe it is any better today.

It became clear to me that not only did we not understand our own profession very well, but the media certainly didn't understand what nursing did, either. State and federal government wasn't far behind. If you look at policy issues and everything surrounding reimbursement and patient care, you'll see that everything revolves around a medical model, and it's difficult to see nursing's role.

The interesting thing is hospitals exist for nursing care. They don't exist for physician care. If patients needed physicians they could go to their office. When patients need a hospital they need nursing care because the physicians aren't there 24 hours per day. But we still think of them as a physician's place and physicians are still the draw.

Nobody goes to a hospital and says, "I'm coming here because Sheryl Stogis is the nurse in critical care and everybody tells me she's the best." They go because Dr. Smith tells them to go and he must be a good doctor, or more likely, because that's what their insurance plan will cover. There's a lot of validity to that but, again, there is nothing past that medical model's conversation. I just don't know how to get past it because nobody understands what we do, and if you don't understand it, you certainly can't place a value on it.

That's why Activity Based Management (ABM) and Process Improvement (PI) methodologies are interesting to me. With ABM we are looking at the amount of time nurses spend on clinical, patient-centered activities versus non-clinical, clerical tasks, and the corresponding costs. When reimbursement was cut, hospitals tried to balance the budget by eliminating positions.

They couldn't fire the nurses because they were still needed. So they laid off clerical support and other non-nursing departments and gave those tasks to nursing, because nurses had to be on the units anyway. How many times have you seen nurses answering the phones while they are busy trying to provide patient care, or completing paperwork for the lab, or trying to track down a snack for a patient who has been off the unit all day, or even transporting a patient from one department to another because the transport team is closed for the evening?

After these problems are identified, Process Improvement approaches can be used to address the problems. Nurses perform many tasks that do not contribute to patient outcomes because hospital administrators and others still don't understand what nurses do. If they did, nurses wouldn't be spending such a small amount of their time on patient education, even though the research says the more education you provide the patient, the better they do in the long run. Instead, nurses are only able to devote their left-over time to patient education, which is typically less than 10% of their day.

Process Improvement methods intrigue me because there is so much that people could do to fix their own jobs if they felt they had permission. It's amazing how we wait until a consultant is hired to tell you what you know you should do, and gives you permission to do it.

On the positive side, there has been public recognition for the value of nursing through the work of Dr. Linda Aiken and a few other prominent nurse researchers. Through their research, the correlation has been made that nurses do impact the outcome of care and patient safety. The question now becomes, "How do we do that?"

Wouldn't you say another way that hospitals are trying to shine the spotlight on nursing is by pursuing Magnet designation?

I have mixed feelings about Magnet status. On one hand, it's educating the public about the value of nursing. That can be a tremendous PR campaign for nursing and the hospital. On the other hand, I struggle with how patients will actually use this information. Are patients choosing a hospital based on nursing care? Are they even making that decision based on their choice of physician? My guess is that they're going with the hospital that is approved by their insurance plan. Of course, if they have a traditional, open plan and they can go anywhere they'd like with the same amount of coverage, then they'll look for the best physician. They might even take into consideration which is the better hospital. And I think they use "good hospital" synonymously with "good nursing care."

I just can't see someone saying they would go out of their system and pay out of pocket in order to choose a Magnet designated hospital over what's covered in their plan. I don't even think there's anything set up in the system to help you choose based on that designation. So, while it's educating the public, we still have a way to go.

Now the interesting thing is I don't think we need Magnet designation or even JCAHO accreditation. This has been my theory all along. These organizations are only asking you to implement and document the things you should be doing anyway. I wrote a book on accreditation and certainly there's value to it if you have no idea what the right things are. If you want to be a good organization you'll be doing those things anyway, so why are you paying a lot of money to have people tell you what I think you already know?

Do you not want medication administration to be error free? I would, and I don't need JCAHO to tell me that. Wouldn't you want a collaborative environment, because that will help retain nurses? I would. That makes sense to me. Does having Magnet designation make my organization more collaborative? I don't know. I think if you have one visionary CEO or CNO who says, "We're just going to do the right things right," you'll probably end up with as good or a better hospital than those with all the correct designations and accreditations.

We have just gone through an election year and the topic of health care is getting a lot of attention. How can nursing influence health policy?

The problem with us [nursing] is that we are our own worst enemies sometimes. We sabotage ourselves. We can't even decide an entry level into practice, and because of that, we have no voice—we have no single voice in this. We don't say this is who we are and this is what we stand for. At least in hospitals, the nursing care is part of the entire "bed" or "room" charge, along with housekeeping and others. I don't see any influential positions addressing nursing other than patient safety-related things, which is a good start, but I sometimes feel like I am back trying to decide what I'd like to do with my career and I am having what I consider to be leaders in nursing tell me, "If you want to be a leader in health care, don't get a degree in nursing."

My husband and I have talked about this for a long time and we believe we're heading towards some kind of defined health care plan for the nation. Right now we have estimates of nearly 46 million Americans who are uninsured, which is significant. The issues on the table will be, "Who will pay for it?" and "How are we going to do it?" That will be the trigger to have a much more serious discussion about what nursing does and how will we pay for nursing. I fully believe that once we enter in those discussions we can no longer have a medical model of care. It must be a patient-centered model of care. That's when nursing starts to say, if we're smart and not arguing about entry level into practice, that if you're talking about patient care, then you're talking about nursing.

But we're still not a player in the political decision-making arena where this happens. We might be a player in patient safety, which is a clinical type issue, but we're not a player overall.

How do we get to be a player?

That's Politics 101. It has to be the right person at the right time in the right setting. There's a philosophy in politics called the open window. It says that when everything comes together—it rarely happens—that is when change occurs. In this instance, we'll need a heightened public awareness that nurses do have a huge impact on care, and we'll need a partner in Congress, or the Senate, or someone who's willing to change federal regulation, which is never an easy thing to do. When these things come together, we'll see a change in nursing and health care.

Maybe the trigger will be having the nation face how we're going to address a national insurance program. Because if it's not set up right, we're going to be in the same bind in 10 years as we are with Social Security. Maybe there will be more open minds and this one little window will open up, and through that window, everything will come together and a big change will occur.

What I would like is to have a nurse as the head of the Department of Health and Human Services—someone who makes policy decisions, who decides reimbursement, and who consults with Congress and the President on where health care should be focused.

Change sometimes takes forever, but you can't even start the process until the discussion begins. Let's start that discussion.

Sheryl L. Stogis, RN, Dr. PH
Assistant Clinical Professor
Department of Public Health, Mental Health and
Administrative Nursing
University of Illinois College of Nursing
Illinois

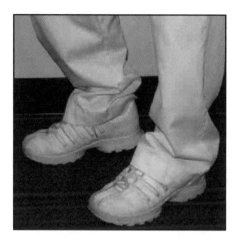

CHAPTER 15

Master Artist

G rowing up, it never entered my mind to become a nurse. When I was very young I wanted to emulate Indiana Jones and become an archeologist. In college I was a psychology major, then I thought of becoming a sociology major or even going into medicine, but after looking at nursing as a career I realized that I could be all of those things. For instance, the love of archeology is uncovering the past and that is one of the techniques I use when working with some of my geriatric patients. Their awareness of the present is unclear, and their awareness of the future is also unclear, but their awareness of the past is often crystal clear and it's my job to uncover that and help them. Nursing is the perfect blend for someone who has multiple interests.

One question I get asked all the time is whether I'm studying to become a doctor, just because I'm a man. I always have to smile and say, "No, I want to be a nurse. This is what I do."

I began my health care career as a nursing assistant in a nursing home that specialized in Alzheimer's care. That was probably the hardest unit. You need to remember that you are caring for people who have lived their entire lifetime being human and there is no reason why that should stop the moment they arrive on your unit. Everyone wants his or her loved ones to be cared for with the utmost dignity.

The progression from nursing assistant to RN is a natural one for many people. After 2 years I transferred to Waukesha Memorial Hospital and graduated from a nursing program. I've been an RN since 1997.

Has nursing lived up to your expectations?

Totally. I was talking with my wife Patty, who's also a nurse, about how rewarding this profession is. Major hospitalization is a milestone in anybody's life and the opportunity to be there and make a difference is extremely rewarding. I never thought it would make me feel as good about being a nurse as it has.

One of my strengths is my sense of humor. It's also one of my weaknesses. I have to learn how to bottle it because there are times when my jokes aren't as funny as I think they are. The patient and I may be laughing hysterically, while another nurse is giving us a smirk thinking, "There's Andre thinking he's clever again!"

Can you give me an example of using humor at work?

This is more a humorous story rather than actually using humor. I was working with a gentleman with advanced cancer who had been hospitalized 4 or 5 times, and each hospitalization required further surgical revisions. We all know that this requires drinking volumes of bowel prep, which tests your fortitude as a patient. He told me that he couldn't stand the taste and absolutely refused to comply. We sat down for a while and he shared his experience of all that he'd been through and I told him that I could make this drinkable for him. I mixed together a number of different beverages but he still couldn't bring himself to drink the concoction.

So, I decided to show him that it was indeed palatable—and started drinking it myself! I drank quite a bit before he finally agreed to give it a try. We sat down and drank the laxative cocktail together. As a matter of fact, he even admitted that it was fairly good tasting! (Now,

I know what you're thinking, and I have to say that I experienced only very mild side effects.) From that point on, every time the gentleman was readmitted he asked for me to be his nurse. We really developed a close relationship.

Is there anything else you'd like to share about being a nurse?

I can't stress enough that the people I work with are the best. I couldn't have handpicked a better group. I also know that becoming a good nurse takes time. Two years of being a nurse does not a master make. Nursing is an art, and to be good at your art you need to practice, and practice takes time. We all aspire to be master artists.

Andre Pells, RN, BSN
Charge Nurse, Medical Surgical Department
Wisconsin

CHAPTER 16

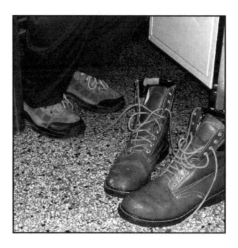

A Message of Hope

I started out as a corpsman in the Navy, and I completed my sea duty with the Marines in 1961. My outfit was the very first to go to Vietnam. We were floating around the South China Sea and got word to go into the Gulf of Tonkin, so we flew up 250 miles and jumped across the Me Kong River into Vietnam. I was there for 8 months when my appendix ruptured and I was flown to our base in Okinawa. I figured I covered all the bases, as I was in the Navy, wearing a Marine Corps uniform, in an Army hospital, and an Air Force surgeon operated on me.

Your journey in nursing has led you to community health work. Tell me about that.

I became a nurse after coming home from Vietnam and eventually became a nurse anesthetist. I enjoyed it, but I wanted more interaction with patients. A friend recommended trying home health nursing. I love it because it involves a lot of teaching and working with families.

I recently worked with a patient who had cancer. Whenever she needed home health nursing, her family would request that I see her. I spent a lot of time with her and her family, and when she passed away the family sent me a very nice card that read in part, "My mom really looked forward to your visits." It was so nice of them to write me a letter at such a sad time. It's this kind of thing that happens every month or two that validates what I am doing and makes me appreciate my work. It's very rewarding

What do you consider to be your most important contribution to patients?

I think that the most important thing to offer someone is hope. I believe patients need someone to listen to them and be honest, regardless of their situation. We have to love the people around us, and do the best we can today.

Is there another experience that illustrates hope?

In 2001, I volunteered with my son and daughter-in-law, who are both OB-GYN physicians, on a medical mission to Malawi, Africa. We set up our practice in their 120-bed hospital that only had 3 or 4 nurses and no doctors. This was the first time my son and I had worked together and he delivered the first baby of 2001. As I was tending to the mother, I looked over the screen and realized this was my son operating. It was a wonderful moment.

Would you consider your work to be heroic?

I don't know that I would use that word. I'm at a point in my life where I can stay home and not work. I work now because I love what I do. The only reason God ever made any of us is to help one another. It doesn't matter who you are, what you do, or what country you live in, sooner or later we're all going to need help. I'm really here to help people.

Tony Beste, RN
Case Manager, Home Health
Illinois

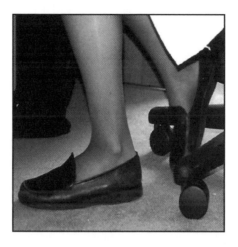

Making a Difference

I've always liked the idea of helping people, but I really wanted to be an airline stewardess when I was growing up. I thought that I would travel the world and meet interesting people. I changed my focus to nursing, but still maintained my initial dream of being able to travel and get a job anywhere in the country—as a nurse.

I've been a nurse for 23 years. I am a critical care nurse who found a niche in the emergency department. As a critical care nurse, I could write my own ticket as far as work flexibility was concerned. You could really work just about anywhere because the job is basically the same. It's just the paperwork and people that are different.

What attracted you to the ER?

I liked the fast pace and the unpredictability, and you see everything there. I really enjoyed that saving the life mode. I had the opportunity and ability to make a difference in someone's life. It's never quite as dramatic as what you see on television, but the content is the same.

The downside is that you never really finish in the ER. You start working with a patient, and then you hand him off to another unit, whether it's the OR, or the ICU. You never really get completion with a patient.

Is there a significant story or event that captures your experience in the ER?

I remember about 10 years ago, one of my peers became my patient.

We received a radio call that a woman was coming in with chest pain. She refused to go to the nearest hospital and requested to come to Ingalls because she was an employee. The paramedics had begun advanced cardiac life support (ACLS) protocol—she had significant chest pain. When she arrived, we had everything in place for her and were arranging for the cardiologist to come in. We were giving her medications and doing everything we could to save her.

As I was looking at her, I saw her heart rate dropping and I knew with every sense of my being that she was dying. I knew that if we didn't act fast, that she would die. I don't know how you know that, but you just do.

We managed to get the cardiologist, and sent her to the cardiac catheterization lab within 20 minutes. She survived and had a regular life after that. It is one of the few times I have had closure with a patient in the ER. It was also one of the most frightening times of my career.

Do you consider your work heroic?

Nurses are really modest people. We do a lot of heroic things, but we have a hard time claiming that.

Gail Ratko, RN, BSN, OCN, CCRP
Clinical Research Coordinator
Illinois

CHAPTER 18

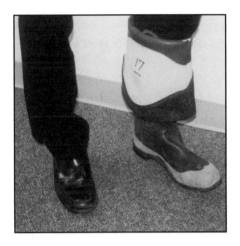

Grace Under Pressure

I joined the volunteer fire department on July 6, 1976. When I spoke to the Fire Chief about the job, he said, "Boy, this stuff's going get in your blood and you're never going be able to wash it out!" He was right. Within a few years I became a paramedic, then a firefighter and an engineer.

Back then, becoming a paramedic was something new and we were taught by nurses. I think they required 24 hours of clinical practice in the ER, and I doubled up and did 48. It was a fantastic experience. I also had a great mentor named Millie Sims—a wonderful southern gal who taught me how to give my very first IM injection. We prepped the patient, and she told me to take the syringe and just throw it like a dart. So I held the syringe and threw it like a dart! After it bounced off the patient, she calmly gave me a clean needle and syringe and told me, "Well that's real fine, but this time, hold it like a dart, and don't let go!" She was wonderful.

My professional goal was to become an EMS (Emergency Medical System) coordinator, but I needed a nursing degree, so I applied to nursing school. At this point, I had also been on the list for the fire department for 2 years. I was going to let fate determine which path my career would take by seeing who would accept me first. Wouldn't you know, fate preferred that I make the decision—I was accepted by both places on the same day. I chose nursing.

You mentioned having a mentor...

I've had several mentors in my career. There was a nurse in the ER, Vince, who taught me so much about being a nurse. He taught me "grace under pressure," and how to be calm and stay in the zone. I remember his words to this day.

The third major mentor in my career was my boss on a telemetry unit, Marian Peters. She was my idol. Not only did she give me very wise advice about my career moves at the hospital, but she also taught me that as a nurse, I should make every move count. She was always there for me to offer support, encouragement, and wisdom.

How do you find your mentors? Not every nurse has been as lucky to work with such nurturing people.

I don't really search them out—they're just there, and I learn from them.

Do you consider yourself a mentor to others?

I try to be. I try to pass along the pearls of wisdom that have made a difference for me.

John Ratko, RN, BSN, EMT-P
Emergency Nurse
Illinois

CHAPTER 19

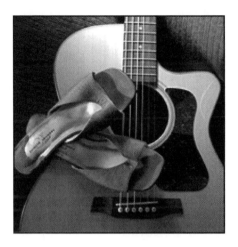

Cheery and Contagious Enthusiasm!

I always wanted to be a nurse. I never questioned it; other than I also secretly wanted to be a choral teacher.

I try to help people feel better. When I was in high school I volunteered to be a Sunshine Geriatric Volunteer at a local nursing home and when my picture came out in their newsletter, they said I had "cheery and contagious enthusiasm!"

I knew I would go into OB the first time I opened my OB textbook. I never thought about a nurse doing something happy. I always thought that nurses only took care of sick people; that all of nursing would be sad, and that I would be giving this great comfort. I never thought about what it would be like to take care of people who were experiencing the happiest time of their lives.

I remember taking care of a woman who already had 5 boys and was ready to deliver her sixth child. She desperately wanted a girl, and the nurses were secretly hoping the same thing. She had a girl via cesarean section, and we wanted to surprise her when she woke up. We wallpapered the ceiling of her room with bath mats covered in pink flamingos that said, "It's a Girl!" When she opened her eyes, she was thrilled. I'm sure she'll always remember it!

What qualities do you think are needed to make a good nurse?

Someone who will go one more step for his or her patient.

You and I have worked together in the past, providing programs to nursing audiences. I've seen nurses laugh and cry when you perform.

And I always promise there will be no sing-alongs! I love sharing my message through music, and I'd like to share the lyrics to one of my songs that really capture the essence of nursing.

Unsung Heroes

This is a song for all the unsung heroes
Who go unnoticed everyday
They're not seeking fame and glory
Though they deserve it anyway
You may not think a simple kindness
Would be worthy of a song
That one person cannot change the world
But my friends
You would be wrong
This is a song for all the unsung heroes
We wrote these words with you in mind
Should you ever think, 'I'm not that special'
Look in the mirror and a hero you will find

© 2004 Deb Gauldin Productions, Inc.

You're a therapeutic humorist and professional speaker. Do you still consider yourself a nurse?

I do. I'm a nurse in every interaction. I still ask, "What is it that you need from me?" That's what a nurse asks. Nurses do serious work, and sometimes forget to lighten up about it. I have a very strong desire to tell other nurses that they're okay; to reaffirm for them that they're valuable and that the work they're doing is important. I don't think nurses realize the importance of their work. I think that the greatest gift you could give to nurses is profound respect for the work they do.

Deb Gauldin, RN, PMS
Speaker, Humorist, Author
North Carolina

CHAPTER 20

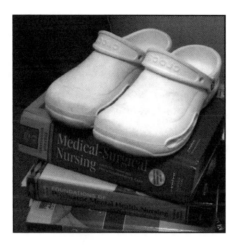

Somebody's Hero

I am nearly finished with my third semester of nursing school, in a 5-semester program. I will graduate with my Associate Degree in Nursing and will be eligible to take the NCLEX exam sometime next year.

How did you decide on Nursing as a profession?

Actually I had already started coursework for a master's in counseling program, but it didn't feel right for me. I have a bachelor's in sociology with a concentration in women's studies and I was thinking about what I wanted to do with my career. I called my mom, who has always been an OB nurse, for advice. I had never voiced it before, but I told her that I wanted to be a midwife, and she gave me great advice because a few of her friends are nurse midwives.

Why didn't you talk to her about your interest in being a midwife when you were growing up, especially since

your mom is a nurse?

I think it was precisely because my mom was a nurse that I wanted to do something entirely different. I wanted to join the Peace Corps or teach women's studies, or do something outside of the box. I think it was one of those rebellious kid things where you refuse to have anything to do with what your parents do.

When I went into women's studies I felt I was part of a strong community and that I could do a lot to help other women. That's probably where the midwifery came from. I was interested in studying women in our society and how they're marginalized, not only by how much money they make, but by their access to health care. I'm very passionate about that. Regardless of whether I eventually do become a midwife, I believe I'll always have a focus on women's health issues.

How did you happen to choose this school of nursing?

I applied at several colleges and universities in Iowa, Illinois, and North Carolina but this program had the first opening. There are enormous waiting lists for nursing school. My mom's alma mater received more than 800 applications for only 200 openings. Baccalaureate programs run a little differently. They accept you as a general student, but you are not allowed to take nursing classes until there is an opening, so it is unclear when you will start the program.

As much as I feel that I should be getting a BSN, I'm glad to be in this program. I already have a baccalaureate degree and I'm excited about the prospect of working as a nurse.

I had to take classes and become a nurse's aide as a prerequisite for this nursing program. That was the first time I had ever worked with patients before and I had so many wonderful experiences. I remember an elderly man who was at risk for falls, and I was with him during much of the day. He held my hand so tightly, and when it was time for me to leave he started crying. It broke my heart. I never felt so needed for not doing anything. I realized that sometimes people just need your presence; they need somebody to care. That made me look at nursing differently. That was a very moving experience.

I'd love to know more about your nursing program and what you're experiencing in your clinical practicum.

It really depends on your instructors. I've had some really fabulous clinical instructors and only one that was not so helpful. Although she's been a nurse for a long time she's a fairly new instructor. I think it will take some time for her to feel comfortable enough to trust the students' clinical practice.

We also work closely with the nurses on the units. There are a couple of fantastic nurses who really enjoy the students and go out of their way to seek us out for different clinical experiences. They'll ask if we'd like to see or participate in certain procedures. But most of the time we feel like we get in the nurses' way. A major criticism we hear is that we take too long to complete assessments, etc. It's all valid, but we're still learning the ropes. I think it takes more than a few days a week after only 3 semesters to have mastered time management skills. It's nice when a nurse acknowledges that we're still students and will say, "I remember the first time I inserted a foley catheter. I was nervous, too, but it's really not that big of a deal."

Have there been any other experiences at school that stand out for you?

I've had some wonderful clinical experiences. The most fun I've ever had was working in OB. Being in labor and delivery was like being in an entirely different world, and most people left the unit happy. It was a completely different atmosphere, and didn't seem as affected by the nursing shortage as the other units. On the other units nurses are so rushed and short-staffed, running in and out of patient rooms. I could definitely see myself working in labor and delivery after graduation.

I also love teaching. I don't know if I'll teach nursing, but I do enjoy patient teaching. I sometimes get nervous, though, when I am explaining something to a patient because I don't know everything. I can imagine my patient thinking, "She has no idea what she's doing," and sometimes I have to agree with them, but most times patients are accepting. They know I am a student nurse and don't mind the fact that I am still learning.

I realize you still have 2 more semesters of school left, but I wonder if you consider any of your actions to be heroic?

(Pause...) Yes, I do actually. I think there are a lot of little things that I've done, not necessarily as a nurse, but as a person, that mean a lot to other people. When you're a nurse, it's considered part of your job, but it's much more than that to the people you care for.

There are also times when I haven't felt heroic. Instead, I felt badly about something I said or did which might not have been the right thing for my patient. I should have been their hero, but I wasn't. Maybe there's an expectation that nurses have that we think we should be somebody's hero.

That's such an interesting way to look at it. I'm really looking forward to seeing how your career unfolds.

Kate Gauldin, BA
Nursing Student
Iowa

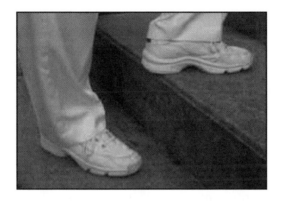

CHAPTER 21

Twice Called

I wanted to be a nurse since I was a little girl. I never dreamed of being anything else. I followed that dream and I've been a nurse for more than 40 years. I was a licensed practical nurse for 22 years before I became a registered nurse. I happened to get married at an early age, and back then they didn't let married women go to nursing school.

I started out delivering babies, and then I worked on a medical-surgical floor. I also worked in the emergency department, and after graduating from college I gained experience in the ICU. That was very challenging.

What drew you to wound care?

About 10 years ago the hospital decided to start a wound clinic, and when they needed another nurse to staff the unit I volunteered. I started out working only 5 hours per week, and now I'm working here 5 days per week.

You are also a parish nurse. Tell me about that.

I had no idea what parish nursing was, but I soon found out that it was a way for nurses to work with the people in their congregations and help them stay healthy. You do that by being an educator, counselor, and advocate. I work at my church on Sunday mornings, where I am available in between services and by phone.

I have also coordinated continuing education programs throughout the hospital on parish nursing. So far I have had more than a dozen classes and more than a hundred graduates. My dream is to have a parish nurse in every church in Decatur.

What motivated you about this type of nursing?

I have always felt that nursing is a calling and, as a parish nurse, you have been called twice. Nurses aren't always encouraged to be spiritual at work, but as a parish nurse it is one of your roles. This isn't traditional hands-on nursing. You're doing what nurses are meant to do, which is treating the mind, body, and spirit.

Would you share some of your experiences?

I work primarily with an older population, but I do have a few high school students who get their blood pressure checked every week. I use that time as an opportunity to talk with them about their grades and their hopes for college.

One of the biggest interventions of parish nursing is presence. You are giving yourself to people, whether you are holding their hands and talking with them, or just sitting in the same room with them. You are connected on their level. You are present with them.

Carol Smith, RN, MS, CWOCN
Enterostomal Therapist
Parish Nurse Coordinator
Illinois

CHAPTER 22

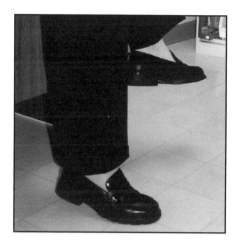

We See Amazing Things

How would you describe College Health nursing?

There is a major difference between what I do and what school nurses do. Surprisingly, we see a little bit of everything here. We have a very diverse student population, with many international students. Most of our students are residents on campus and are away from home for the first time. They're working through adjustment issues ranging from homesickness and culture shock to dealing with having a roommate. What we see here is what you would see in the community.

Would you share some of your experiences?

We see some amazing things here. We had a student who had muscular dystrophy and was in a motorized wheelchair, who came in every day during his lunch break so that we could help him with his bowel program.

We have another student who was diagnosed with cancer a few months ago. She's on chemotherapy and trying to stay in school. She comes in every day for injections to help boost her red blood cells. She is so incredibly strong. Not only is she doing well, but she is also helping us understand the process she is going through—emotionally and physically.

Do you work solely with students?

Actually, we also see the staff and employees. Not too long ago I saw a woman in first degree heart block. You have to have excellent assessment skills, and you have to be able to make decisions and work independently.

What gives you the most satisfaction as a College Health nurse?

My summers off! I paid my dues in the hospital working all shifts and holidays. Now I work 9 AM-5 PM, Monday through Friday, from August 15 to May 15—with vacation time thrown in the middle.

The most rewarding part of my job during those 9 months is the opportunity to do one-to-one teaching and wellness education. I love this age group! It's wonderful to have students come back to me and say that they did something because they remembered what I had told them. It's nice to know that they've been listening all along.

Barbara Allanach, RN, C
Director of Student Health Services
Illinois

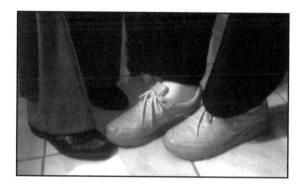

The Leg Bone's Connected to the....

A conversation with Linda Polzin, RN, BSN, about her mother, Marian Tylk, RN.

Linda, do you remember any of the stories your mom told you when you were growing up?

She has a lot of great stories! She was a nurse and worked for several years before taking time off to raise her family. She didn't go back to work until I was 10 or 11 years old. Most of her stories were about how much health care had changed while she was away.

This is one of my favorites:

My mom was working at the hospital one evening when a doctor called and wanted the lytes checked on his patient. My mom proceeded to call maintenance to come and check out the overhead lights. The maintenance man came and inspected the lights, and told my mom that everything was fine. So, my mom called the doctor to tell him that the lights were absolutely fine.

When he asked her what they were, she said, "When you turn the switch up, they go on, and when you turn the switch down, they go off."

He was a very good person. He got a little chuckle out of it, and then explained to her what electrolytes were.

That was very kind of him! Are there any other stories that show how much health care has changed since your mom became a nurse?

I remember a story that she told about body parts. When she was in nursing school, she had to carry a leg down the stairs to the incinerator—not to pathology mind you—but to the incinerator. They amputated a patient's leg, wrapped it in paper, and asked her to dispose of it!

Can you imagine?

I can only imagine what future generations will think of us...

Marian Tylk, RN
Retired
Class of '38
Illinois

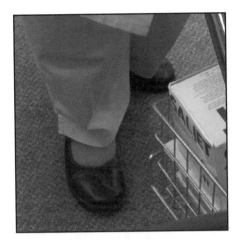

CHAPTER 24

Unwritten Benefit

W hen I worked in oncology, research was valued because it gave people another option, another way of addressing their situation. It was a benefit for them.

How is that option presented when a person comes to a teaching hospital with a diagnosis of breast cancer?

At our hospital, when a patient first comes in to see the breast cancer doctor, they often have an appointment at the Breast Cancer Clinic. Here they see a medical oncologist who specializes in breast cancer, a breast surgeon, and a radiation oncologist who specializes in breast cancer. At this visit they do what's called staging. They identify exactly where this person is in her disease process. They review all of the patient's diagnostic tests, pathology results, mammograms, lab tests, tumor measurements, and then the doctors have a better understanding of what's happening and start to make a plan with the patient and her family. Sometimes the plan is to do surgery first, then chemo, followed by radiation. Sometimes chemo is offered first, then surgery, then back again for chemo.

I worked with a team of doctors and generally the entire team is involved with different research projects.

Are patients ever steered toward a specific research project?

They are offered various options in their treatment plans, and often a research study may be a part of them. All of the research studies are specific and not everyone would qualify for every study. It's often overwhelming for the patients, their families and friends at the time, but if they show an interest in a study, I come in and meet with them so they can put a face with my name. I review the highlights of the study and review the Informed Consent with them, and give everyone (spouses, friends) a copy of the consent. I tell the patient that I'll call her in a few days and arrange for a visit within a week to further discuss the study. I encourage everyone to read the consent and write down every question as it occurs to them. If they see something they don't understand, they should write it right there on the consent form, so that when we're going over it in person they'll know that it'll be addressed.

It's much better than having them write their questions on a separate sheet of paper which they inevitably forget to bring with them. This way, everyone's questions are answered. And if I can't answer them, I'll get in touch with the doctor. But by and large, I'll have the answers for them when it comes to the research study.

Is this usually done by the research nurse?

Yes, it's better to do that with a nurse rather than a research aid or a research coordinator. You don't have to be a nurse to be a research coordinator, but I believe that's a role for a nurse. I can't see how a nurse wouldn't want to work in research. It's so interesting. You can be such a strong patient advocate, and nurses need to assume those roles.

Nurses see the big picture. They understand the clinical issues and how to approach the patient to ease their fear. If it's a new diagnosis, that patient is experiencing absolute fear. They're going to take a drug, chemotherapy, which will do a lot of things to their body. Besides the nausea, vomiting, and hair loss, their tongue and nails could turn black, their skin could break out like they were 15 years old, it's amazing what some of these chemotherapy drugs can and will do. But you have to have someone there who understands this and who can explain how these drugs will affect their bodies.

As a research nurse, you do a lot of patient teaching, and it begins with explaining what a research study is. What do you think of when you hear the word research? Quite a few people associate research with guinea pig. They think they're just being used in an experiment. But I try to reassure them and say things like, "We're actually looking at 15,000 people from across the country or throughout the world in this study," or, "These drugs are all FDA approved. What we're looking at is using a different combination or different dosing for this regimen. We're not giving you something that will hurt you."

I also tell them that they will have me as their nurse. They'll have the treatment room nurse, and they'll get to know us both, but I'll be another set of eyes and ears for them. I'll be just a phone call away. Once I have a patient on my study and she signs the consent, I give her my card, and on the back I have my cell phone number. So if patients have questions or concerns while they're not here, they can reach me. I really want to know if they're going to have problems on a Saturday afternoon.

Did you get a lot of calls?

Not really, no. And the calls that I got, I needed to get. One of those calls was from a patient receiving chemotherapy. She had the doctor's number, but she couldn't understand the hospital phone system. I'm glad she called me because that occurred on a weekend. I was able to reach the doctor and the patient was admitted to the hospital. She was really dehydrated and by Monday she would have gotten much worse.

I had another patient who had flown to Washington, DC on business. I was working on a GI research project then and he was in the study. He called me from DC and told me he was bleeding. He didn't know what to do, but he knew that he couldn't fly home. I told him he needed to go to the hospital, but he didn't want to go. "Trust me," I said, trying to lighten the mood, "I don't want you to go either. It's more paperwork for me!"

This was the day before Thanksgiving, I was in a Borders parking lot, and it was raining, but I stayed on the phone with him until I could convince him to go to the hospital. He finally listened to me and, as it turned out, he was there for a week.

So as a research coordinator, it sounds as if you function like a case manager.

More like a case manager for the study. I make sure that they complete their paperwork, understand what they have going on, and I shepherd them through the system. If they need an MRI, I make sure it gets done. I have enough connections to make it happen pretty quickly.

So, if patients decline to participate in the research study, are they left to deal with all of these services on their own?

They fend for themselves primarily. They'll see a doctor and the treatment nurse, and all of the same services are available to them, if prescribed by the doctor, but they often have to make all the arrangements on their own.

In oncology nowadays, there are a lot of resources available for patients. Every oncologist has his or her treatment center, and within the treatment center there are very qualified nurses. But you know, the patients are there for a short time period, and the nurses are busy. The patients still receive attention, but in a research study, they'll get a little more.

Are there any other benefits to being in a study?

Besides the opportunity to try new treatments and therapies, the only benefit that is identified on the informed consent is written as, "contributing to the good of mankind." Some don't really call that a benefit. But I tell them, "And you get me." That's the unwritten benefit.

What kinds of questions do you get from people who are considering being in a study?

The biggest question has to do with FDA approval of a drug. The study may say that this drug is not FDA approved but it actually is. What's not approved is that particular application in a different regimen. There are drugs that are approved for lung cancer that we're now using in breast cancer treatment. So, it's not FDA approved for use in breast cancer but we're looking at it as a targeted therapy that's going to stop the blood supply to this tumor. The bottom line is it's not FDA approved for that application.

There are also a lot of blinded studies, which are done in such a way that the patients (single-blinded), or patients and their doctors (double-blinded), do not know which drug or treatment is being given. (The opposite of a blinded study is an open label study.) We want to make sure that the results are not affected by a placebo effect.

There aren't too many blinded studies in oncology, but just about all of them were in GI. In those studies, the patient might be given a placebo and I explain to the patient that it is a non-therapeutic pill, a "sugar" pill, or a pill without any active ingredients.

The placebo studies are a little more difficult. When a patient enters the study, they're generally at their wits' end about their disease. They're looking for an answer and they're willing to participate—even in a blinded study—to find that answer.

It's a little harder on me as well because I tend to watch these patients a little more closely. If I haven't heard from them in a week I'll call to see how they're doing, check on their side effects. That's what you're looking for, adverse effects.

So I'll call and ask, "Anything going on?"

"No," they say.

"Any changes?" I ask again.

"Oh, I feel good." But then there's the Hawthorne affect. People get on a study and they think they're doing great. Just like that gentleman who called me from Washington, DC. He felt that he was fabulous. He knew he was receiving the "real" drug. He just knew it. And that's why he decided to fly out to Washington for a meeting.

But I didn't want him to fly. I didn't know if he was taking a placebo or if he was on the medication, but I was concerned. People believe that they're getting the drug, and they believe they're getting better. The mind is very powerful. As it turned out, this patient wasn't taking the drug. We had to get him un-blinded because of his adverse effects and we needed to notify the treating physician in the DC hospital. It was a critical situation.

What was the best case scenario that you experienced as a research nurse?

Very simply, it is when the patient gets better. It's also very exciting to see an actual project, or a drug come to market. That's so encouraging. Sometimes in a study you'll find that people are responding to the treatment and they've completely turned around. You can call the sponsor, the drug company manufacturing the drug being studied, and request that they do a "special needs" for the patient, which allows the patient to continue taking the drug. This usually happens when they're getting good outcomes and think the drug might go to market soon.

I strongly encourage people to go to a medical center if they've been diagnosed with a serious illness. Go a scientist, a medical doctor who actually does his or her own research. These studies may be part of what they could offer to you as part of your treatment plan. You owe it to yourself to research that doctor's scientific background and go to someone who knows their specialty.

That's the answer for the future; otherwise you're just doing usual and customary. There are so many new things happening in health care, so many advances, and having someone who's on top of things in research is definitely to your advantage.

Can you share some examples of studies that you've worked on?

There was a very interesting study that was looking at how physical stress manifests in colon tissue. The doctor's theory was on leaky gut syndrome. The subjects (the people who participated in the study), were both healthy volunteers and people with disease. It was so interesting to see the results of this project.

At the start of the study the doctor took a colon tissue sample from each of the study subjects to use as the baseline, and for 5 consecutive days the subjects would come in and submerge their hands in an ice bath. The ice was the physical stressor. On the first day it was only for a minute, and by the end of the week, their hands were in ice for 30 minutes. At the end of the study, they'd have another tissue sample taken from the lower portion of their colon.

The stress on the colon was incredible. It was simply amazing to see what happened to those tissue samples. They actually shrunk with repeated stress, and you could see how the toxins could easily seep out of the colon into the bloodstream.

So when I talk with patients, especially in oncology, I'm very aware of the circumstances they've been in when first diagnosed with this devastating illness. Many times I'll hear that a spouse had been laid off, or a parent had been ill or has died, or they've lost their job, or their house. I think about that study and remember how those toxins were released after the body had been exposed to stress. And now they're here, with more stress. Makes you wonder.

Everyone needs to address stress right away. Do your best to get rid of the stress in your life. Meditate, take a yoga class, or take a walk during lunch. Just dump the stress. You don't need to carry it with you.

That's so interesting. It makes me wonder about all the stress we're currently living with. We're in a recession,

people are losing their jobs and their homes, gas prices are fluctuating, and so many millions of Americans don't have health insurance. What is that kind of stress doing to the health of our population?

I'm sure something will come up for many people, just wait. Give it a year after everything settles and I'm sure we will see a lot of people getting sick with some autoimmune disorder. This hasn't been brought up yet, but it will. You know, more women are diagnosed with an autoimmune disorder than men.

If you've been diagnosed with a major illness, ask yourself what happened in the last year or 6 months. What pushed your gut over the limit? My theory is, and I'm just a nurse, but my theory is that these toxins seep through the walls of your gut. They're natural bacteria, but they belong in the colon where they serve a purpose. Instead, the stress that you experience pushes those toxins into your bloodstream, and they travel to whatever area is most predisposed to illness.

Your Achilles' heel...

Yes. And that is where genetics comes in. We're just learning more about obesity and how it may be stress-induced. It's not just overeating; it's what your body does with the food you eat when you're stressed. Diabetes, hypertension, Multiple Sclerosis, Crohn's Disease, ulcerative colitis, cancer—they are all examples of the body attacking its own cells.

Granted, your environment has contributed something, but whatever you're predisposed to, stress will open the door and cause the inflammatory cascade to begin. And along with the inflammatory cascade, cancer cells start to develop, or the myelin sheaths are destroyed in your neurological system, or your insulin process isn't working as it should. The process starts, the inflammatory cascade just rolls, and then you're sick.

You have to take care of yourself. Do not get stressed. It's not worth it. Nurses don't take time out for themselves, but they should. We should know better. Our managers should know better, and should encourage healthy work habits.

Perhaps more hospitals should provide stress reduction programs for their staff?

Besides the once-a-year nurse's week event with massage therapists in the lobby? But seriously, some employers do offer reimbursement for complementary and alternative medicine (CAM) treatments within their benefits packages. I think that's a start.

You've done so much work with oncology patients. Do you have a patient who stands out for you?

I've worked with a lot of patients, and in oncology the experiences are much more intense. I remember one day when I was sitting in the lobby in tears with one of my patients. She came in for her third treatment cycle of chemotherapy.

When I first met Julie, what I noticed first about her was her beautiful, long black hair. I remember telling her to consider cutting her hair before starting the chemo, to a style similar to a wig she would wear once she lost her hair.

"I know it's hard," I told her, "but you're most likely going to lose your hair. Getting it cut short now will give you time to adjust to it. It won't be so much of a shock to you when you start your chemo and you do lose your hair. You could maybe even have a wig made from your own hair. I hate to say it this way," I continued, "but it's easier on you seeing short hairs on your pillow versus the long hair." I told her too that her scalp would probably hurt a lot more when her long hair started falling out. It breaks off and the scalp is very tender.

After you take your first treatment you're still feeling pretty good. With your second treatment you notice the hair loss even more, depending on the drugs, and you are really starting to feel the side effects. The nausea is contained nowadays with better medication, but some people still slip through. By the third treatment, though, fatigue is setting in and the patients don't have the energy like they used to. I tell my patients that they should have someone come to the hospital with them because we won't let them drive after the treatment. The mixture of medications just knocks them out.

So when I came down to the lobby I was surprised to see Julie was there all alone. I walked up to her and asked where her husband was.

"Oh," she smiled, "he's gone away on vacation." It was a trip he had planned with his friends before she was diagnosed with breast cancer. She wanted him to go because, "of all that he's gone through."

"Okay," I replied, hesitatingly, "and who's with you?"

"My friend is picking me up. She's going to meet me downstairs."

Suddenly, I'm seeing flashes of warning lights. There are several problems here. Number one, her husband isn't here, but I can't really blame him because Julie encouraged him to take the trip. I can picture the whole scenario: Julie is feeling guilty because of her diagnosis and so she wants her husband to enjoy a trip that was already planned. She's reassuring Joe that she'll be fine while he's away, and besides her friend will be with her.

But in essence, that friend being with her really meant that her friend would be meeting her downstairs, after the chemo treatment.

Julie has sisters. She has a mother. "Why," I wonder, "isn't her family with her?" Somebody is not accepting this. And she still had her long hair. So, we started talking in the lobby and I asked about her hair.

"Oh, my scalp is killing me," she said, gingerly touching her head.

"But we talked about that. Why haven't you cut your hair?"

"Because my mom told me that I wasn't going to lose my hair."

I told her that I'm sure her mother wanted to believe that she wasn't going to lose her hair, but because her scalp was hurting so badly it was a sign that she was, in fact, losing it. And she confirmed that she was seeing a lot of hair on her pillow and in her comb. I told her to just get it cut short. One less thing to worry about or deal with.

We talked more about her mom and I asked, "Does anybody hug you?"

And now she began to cry, "No. Nobody hugs me anymore."

They don't want to feel the missing breast. "You have to hug them," I told her, and now we're both crying. "You have to let them know you're the same person. You didn't change. You didn't go away." It was tough.

There must have been 70 people in that lobby but we didn't care. I stayed with her for the entire time she was there, and at the end of the day I walked her downstairs to her friend's car.

Her friend wasn't working that day, and didn't have any other plans, so she could have easily stayed with Julie. There was a lack of communication and denial among her friends and family. Julie also needed to allow people to help her. I offered to talk to them for her, but she said that she would have a heart-to-heart with everyone. That visit was a real turning point for her.

Things were much better the next time I saw her. She had cut her hair, and by the following treatment it was all gone, but she had her family by her side from that moment on.

You're such a strong patient advocate. Do you ever need to get involved with your patient's insurance companies?

Yes, I'll go to bat for them but I've never experienced chemo being denied. I know there are cases but I haven't personally seen it.

I run into trouble obtaining coverage for medications to keep your white blood cell count in check during chemotherapy. There's one drug that calls for an injection once a day, and another that's given weekly. The daily injections are less expensive, but let's look at quality of life. Who would prefer to have a daily injection over one that's given weekly?

The insurance companies approve the daily injections, but the fact still remains that the weekly injections, at over $1000 per dose, are still extremely expensive. We're controlled by the pharmaceutical industry, and the insurance companies. It gives me fear constantly if, and when, I change insurance policies.

I had another patient who was 8 years post her diagnosis of breast cancer. Her tumor tissue was HER-2 positive, so she needed to take tamoxifen every day. She was doing pretty well and had been taking her medication consistently over the years. Her insurance carrier had changed and she found out that the new company had a different generic brand in their formulary and this was the only brand they covered.

She started on this brand and was soon complaining of diarrhea. She hadn't had this kind of problem since she started with her treatment 8 years ago.

So, I called the insurance company, and I went all the way up to the head of pharmacy. I tried to explain that her symptoms were specific to this brand of medication, not the type of medication. The brand that she had been taking was manufactured in Israel and the current brand that they used was made in Canada. I told them that the Canadian manufacturer was probably using a different compounding agent that was giving her diarrhea.

I finally got approval from them to cover the former brand of tamoxifen, but it took many phone calls and skilled negotiation.

But when we complain about insurance companies, we forget that someone had to select the companies' level of coverage. Someone made that determination about what tier of medications would be covered, and at what percentage. It goes back to your employer. This is their cost saving measure.

I had an experience with a patient whose insurance policy didn't cover one of her treatment regimens. When I contacted the insurance case manager, they told me that the employer had made that decision and struck it from the policy. No doubt it was a cost saving measure. So, I contacted the employer and asked the HR benefits representative if they were aware of this particular omission. Her answer astounded me.

She knew about the cut and said, "But not too many people were using it."

"Well, what about those few who do?" I asked.

I called my patient, and told her what her husband's employer was doing to cut costs and how it was affecting their health care benefits. I told her to tell her husband to tell the union and anyone else who would listen.

The best part about this was the patient called me about 3 months later and said the union was able to change the policy.

This seems an appropriate time to ask if you consider your work to be heroic.

I guess I am a hero. How many lives did I change with that phone call? I like knowing that my being there for my patients is a good thing.

Linda Polzin, RN, BSN
Senior Research Coordinator
Illinois

SECTION THREE

"Nurture your mind with great thoughts;
To believe in the heroic makes heroes."

Benjamin Disraeli (1804 – 1881)

CHAPTER 25

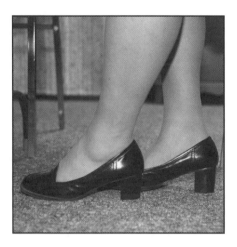

Making a Difference
For Nurses

I just had lunch the other day with some of my classmates. We graduated in 1960 from UW Madison. That was when there were very few schools offering a baccalaureate degree in nursing. But I didn't go for that reason. I went because I wanted to go to college, and I value the education I got there every single day.

It took us 5½ years to get our BSN. For the first 2 years we stayed in the regular dorms and took general classes. Then we moved to the nurses' dorms and took 3 years of clinical coursework. During the final 6 months we chose to specialize in either public health or ward management teaching. I specialized in public health because I thought I would hate teaching, but it turns out I've been teaching all my life.

Tell me about your teaching experiences.

This is really dating me, but one of my very first jobs was teaching people how to survive in bomb shelters. I worked at the VA Hospital

111

in Madison because back then the VA recognized degrees and paid differently. It's there that I learned I loved teaching. It started with patient teaching and progressed to teaching other nurses.

I enjoy creating an environment where other people can grow. You know the old adage that you gain power by giving away control? I think that's true. The more control you give to the people around you the more powerful you are.

I see leaders who are so afraid—no, they are not leaders—I see managers who are so afraid to have anybody know more than they do. That limits you to whatever your body of knowledge is. There is a real difference between a manager and a leader. A leader creates an environment of opportunity for others.

I can remember when I was a nursing administrator, and the first time I helped someone grow. I groomed her.... and she left! I felt so badly for myself. I couldn't understand why she would leave, but afterward I realized that is what leadership is all about. If you are going to run a good organization you don't want the same people staying there forever anyway. It's always hard to lose a good employee, someone you've nurtured along the way. But after a while, you realize it's healthy for the organization and you will groom and nurture the next person as well.

You've always been a strong nurse advocate, and over the past 20 years you've had an incredible opportunity to write and publish a newspaper for nurses in Wisconsin and neighboring states. How did your newspaper, *NURSINGmatters*, get its start?

I've always kept a new business venture file, and I've always thought about doing more for the profession. I felt that I had my administrative job under control, so I began a continuing education and consulting business called, Nursing Productions of America Inc (NPA). I was also on a committee addressing a shortage of nurses in Wisconsin. Funding was running out and I thought that this would be the perfect opportunity for NPA to take this message about the nursing profession to the public.

My good friend and colleague Vivien DeBack, herself a dynamic nursing leader, arranged for me to meet Kevin Smith, who ran *NursingSpectrum* at that time. He said that he'd help me start my nursing publication but he'd like 51% of the business. I told him, "Kevin, I'm too old to work as hard as I know I'll have to for 49% of the business," and that ended our negotiation. *NURSINGmatters* was the result, and we've been dedicated to publishing a newspaper exclusively for nurses for nearly 20 years.

For 6 months we had 4 people working long hours each evening putting together a business plan. I had never done anything like this before, and while I thought it would be difficult for a woman to get a business loan, I didn't realize it was nearly unheard of for a woman to get a bank loan for a publishing business. But, we conducted a market survey and put together a beautiful plan and took it to 6 banks, 5 of which summarily dismissed us.

With the sixth bank, I used the 'good old boy' technique. I had a neighbor from across the hall who knew someone from the bank. It turned out he knew the bank president. So I called and made an appointment, showed him my business plan, and we were given the loan.

I was involved in an entrepreneurial group at the time and I had mentioned that I had been approved for this business loan to start a publishing company for nurses, and they couldn't believe it. They told me that it was a huge accomplishment for a woman. Remember, this was back in 1990. The bank officer also said that only 5% of the people who come in for a loan have a business plan. That amazed me. As nurses we know in order to implement something, you need an assessment and you need a plan, and that's part of the nursing process. That process takes you all through life. You can have a vision but without a plan how can you carry it out? And in order to have a plan, you have to complete an assessment. That piece of my nursing education has served me well in everything I've done.

What changes have you seen in nursing leadership over the years?

I see a struggle for power, particularly in the hospital setting. It's among all departments, not just nursing. Everybody wants a piece of the action. I think hospitals worked more efficiently back when nuns were administrators. They were nuns/nurses first and administrators second. They understood their major product. I don't think hospitals today understand their major product—which is nursing care.

The only reason we need hospitals is because people need nursing care. But while it's their major product, it's not the money-maker. Nursing is part of the room rate.

To complicate matters, let's factor in today's nursing shortage. Try and tell a hospital not to admit patients when they don't have enough nurses on staff. There are very few where nurses call the shots in terms of patient admissions.

So other hospitals still admit patients regardless of how well staffed they are?

Oh absolutely. California has mandated nurse-to-patient staffing ratios. But staffing ratios are not the be-all, end-all because there are so many other variables. You have to consider the physical plan, the age of your nurses, the experience of your nurses, and the acuity of the patients.

I see a trend emerging in nurses becoming credentialed in leadership. Organizations are sending their top level nurses to programs sponsored by the Robert Wood Johnson Foundation and the Wisconsin Organization of Nurse Executives, and others, but I'm not seeing many mid-level managers attending, or staff nurses.

And then I look at hospitals seeking the ANCC Magnet designation, and I think for a lot of them it's a top-down decision. They're doing what they have to do in order to obtain the designation, but there are a significant number of staff nurses who work in these organizations who are saying, "We don't have the power they say we do."

With every right there is responsibility, and I'm not sure if nurses are grabbing onto the responsibility and saying, "Yes, I will act like a nurse leader and I will do what it takes to create an environment where nurses can truly practice nursing."

One of the reasons I support universal health care is that people are finally realizing that nurses work on the wellness end of the spectrum.

If you ask me about my vision for nursing it would be for nurses to become the gate keepers. I go to a nurse practitioner for my health care needs and I haven't seen a doctor since I've gone to her. But I think that if we really want to keep the people in this nation as healthy as they can possibly be, the first contact with the health care system should not be when they're ill.

We should be asking, "How can we keep you healthy?" A system that would be much more economical and have much better outcomes would be one in which everybody had a nurse practitioner. Not everyone will comply, and I don't think you can eradicate all diseases, but I do think that we would have a much better quality of life in a system where we're viewed as a whole person.

We wait until people have had their spirits broken or their emotions broken and eventually it comes out in their body, and then they enter the system. I believe that nurses do the healing, not the curing, and that if we healed some of those emotional and spiritual wounds early on, we wouldn't have to worry about them coming out physically.

I know that a portion of our population uses the Emergency Department as a primary source for health care and many times they don't seek care until they are in crisis.

But that is because of our insurance system. In this country we're spending twice as much per capita on health care as any other country. If you have money and you need good care, you can get it; but if you don't have money, you won't get it. Where are our outcomes on an international basis? According to the World Health Organization, the United States is ranked 37th out of 191 countries, below Saudi Arabia, Morocco, Australia, and even Costa Rica.[1] What is wrong with this picture?

My vision is to have universal health care and have nurses recognized for their value. I also believe that we cannot do that graduating people in 2 years. The more I think about it, the more I think you need a master's degree to practice in this profession. And when you talk about leadership, we haven't stepped up to the plate, have we?

---

[1] World Health Organization, *The World Health Report 2000 – Health Systems: Improving Performance* (Geneva: WHO, 2000).

I think individual leaders need to step up to the plate and accept responsibility for the profession. They need to paint a vision and work to get there, just like Florence Nightingale did.

Besides Florence Nightingale, who are our nurse leaders?

That's exactly part of our problem. They'll probably tell you Florence but nobody since. Look at the Vivien DeBacks of the world. She worked on the national implementation project back in the 70s and she is from Wisconsin. She's very active politically and brings nursing issues into a community perspective. A leader does not necessarily need to be confined to nursing. I serve on a variety of boards for that very reason, so I can talk about the value nursing brings to a society.

It's amazing how little people understand about nurses, but if you can tell a story you'll grab their attention. I don't think we tell our stories enough. That is one of the reasons why I started the newspaper. We have to honor one another and tell one another our stories.

When you talk to politicians about health care, they are asking for stories. They want to hear those individual situations where people didn't have health insurance and what happened as a result. They want the stories. They don't want a generic "we're in trouble without health care" line. Those individual stories carry much weight. Nurses should be proud enough and convinced enough of what they do that they would tell their stories, and recognize one another.

I've been very encouraged because when I started this paper we really had to work for articles. Now, there are so many nurses who are approaching me with their articles, and I feel good about that. They're beginning to see that this is a vehicle where they can get their word out. I receive more articles from staff nurses, though, than from nurse leaders.

What can we do to improve nursing leadership?

Let me give you an example about what's really discouraging for me, and it has to do with leadership. A few years ago there was a hospital nurse who was working with a 16-year-old pregnant girl. The nurse had worked 12 hours the day before, slept at the hospital, got up, and started her shift at 7 AM. Around noon her patient was getting ready to deliver, and a Penicillin IV was ordered. She was also scheduled to have an epidural. The nurse had gone to get the epidural—which they are not supposed to do—but the anesthesiologist or the nurse anesthetist wanted everything ready. In the meantime somebody came in and dropped off the Penicillin. The nurse picked up the wrong medication and gave the epidural— not the Penicillin—and the patient immediately went into convulsions. They saved the baby but lost the mother.

You can imagine the tragedy. The nurse was completely distraught and was sent immediately to the psych ward. Ultimately, she was accused of a felony and was fired. If a nurse can be accused of a felony for a mistake, where's the hazard pay?

What I take issue with is how the nursing administrator handled this incident. She wouldn't allow the nurse to come back to the hospital or talk with the other nurses. She was never given a chance, and she had been an excellent nurse. I realize the gravity of the situation, but where is the nursing leadership in this case? This nurse had made some decisions she shouldn't have and one of them was that she shouldn't have been working so many hours. But, she was a single parent with several children to raise and she was working too much.

The hospital shouldn't have allowed the extra overtime but there is a shortage of nurses and this is a short-term solution. Right after it happened though, there was an acknowledgment section in the newspaper that actually listed the number of extra hours these 3 or 4 nurses had worked in the last quarter.

My point is that leaders have to stand up for nurses. At about the same time as that incident, 3 newborns died after 5 neonatal ICU nurses in Indiana gave the wrong dose of Heparin. But those nurses were treated very differently. The hospital administrator stood behind those nurses. If you're a true leader then you'll stand up for your nurses in good times and bad.

What would you have done differently in that situation?

I would've stood up for the nurse. You know it's a mistake, and you don't fire people for mistakes. Just look at what that does to the rest of the nurses. I would have stood up for her and if they hadn't listened to me I would have resigned.

When I was working as an administrator years ago, I had a nurse who was quoted in our local newspaper as saying that nurses were earning the same salaries as bus drivers. This is dating me, but at the time it was a scandalous story. My administrator called me and said, "We can't have this. You have to fire her." Well, I went down to my office, called my husband and said, "I'm resigning from my job today," and told him the story. He agreed with me and so I went back to my administrator and said, "If you tell me I have to fire her, I'll fire her. But I want you to know you'll have my resignation also because I don't believe that what she did was that wrong."

As a leader you have to be willing to accept responsibility. I know nurses make mistakes but you have to support them. You have to stand up for what you believe, and not let somebody else tell you that you must do something that you know isn't right. You have to have a belief and it can't be, "I believe I can be a nursing administrator." It has to come from inside.

What made you decide to pursue a leadership position?

It was just a fluke! I was working as a staff nurse and the nursing administrator was on extended sick leave. I can remember coming to work one night and saying, "This place is going to the dogs." And then I thought, "Oh my god, maybe that person really does do more than just sit up there in an ivory tower." And so I took a job as an assistant director for the summer. In the fall I decided I had to go back to school. I thought that as one nurse I can make a difference for "x" number of patients, but maybe in a position of greater authority, I can make a difference for even more patients. I wasn't even thinking at that point about making a difference for nurses, but that evolved. If you want nurses to take good care of patients, you've got to take good care of nurses.

What has been your greatest accomplishment to this point in your career?

It has to be the newspaper. I had to learn so many different things. I had never written a business plan before, I had to deal with a banker, and I had to learn a whole new language in the publishing business. I had to work with printers who laid out galleys for us. It's so much easier now with computer software programs, but back then cutting and pasting was done literally.

I also love encouraging people to write articles. I sit on many of these nursing committees for that very reason. At every meeting I'll find someone who will write an article for me. This past election year we focused a great deal of our attention on the campaigns.

For years I've heard nurses say, "Oh, I don't get involved in politics." I think that's changing a little. I think nurses are beginning to see that if we really want to make changes in our practice and our settings, we have to get involved politically.

If you had an opportunity to sit down with the president of the United States, what would you say?

I would say, unequivocally, that a nation is only as healthy as the health of all its people, not just its wealthy ones. I would also show the president some of the waste that's going on in our system. And then I would say, "The people that are equipped to provide the very best health care are nurses. Health care. Not illness care. Let's get people healthy and keep them healthy and then it won't cost us so much."

I'm the first to admit that if we transition to universal health care, it will cost a heck of a lot initially because we have tens of millions of people in this country who haven't been receiving any health care at all. We're looking at a program that's probably not going to be cost effective for 20 years.

But we can't make decisions based on cost alone. Look at how the lack of health care affects the productivity of our workforce, or how drug addictions affect society. We need nurses to work with those people.

I remember talking to a nurse a few years ago and I encouraged her to write an article about her work. She ran a small clinic in an apartment complex that was in a very poor neighborhood. There was one young lady who stood out for her. She said this young girl, who was already the mother of three, would visit and spend time with her in the clinic. One day the girl told her, "You kept me from getting pregnant again. Thank you."

Think about what that does for society.

The other thing I'd say to the president is, "Money doesn't trump everything. Look at what nurses prevent, instead of just seeing what doctors cure."

I'd tell the president a lot, mainly because I love this profession. I have a very deep admiration for nursing and what it can contribute to society. I think I've gained more from this profession than I have ever given back. I have worked with people at their most vulnerable times, and they've been willing to open their souls to me. How many people have had that kind of experience? It's a privilege.

Kaye Lillesand, MSN, RN
Editor, Health Care Consultant
Wisconsin

CHAPTER 26

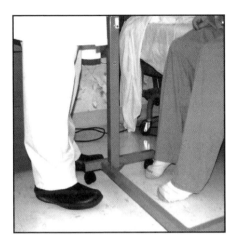

Driven by Compassion

I went into nursing with a lopsided view of what nursing meant. I saw nursing as peripheral to the core of health care; it was a nicety to be loving and compassionate. Imagine that! Now I know that nursing is driven by compassion. We are loving, we are compassionate, but we also have the knowledge and experience to create, implement and evaluate the life-saving techniques and technology that foster healing. Compassion is the medium by which we're able to do that.

I came to live by the word when I heard my patients say, "I need you to help me. My life has been saved, but the quality of my life has been broken. You're the person I trust to make it better."

What is your vision of nursing in the next 20 years?

We're definitely in a crisis, and the crisis is bigger than just the fact that there aren't enough empathetic, scientifically-based nurses to fill these vacancies. Let's empower nurses by publicly recognizing what we do. There is no Oprah out there communicating this fact to consumers. We need a national spokesperson.

What do we do until then?

We need to somehow communicate to the public what the nursing shortage means to health care, and what the consequences are to the consumer.

We also need to provide good care.

Henry Ecker, BS, RN, C
Subacute Director
Illinois

CHAPTER 27

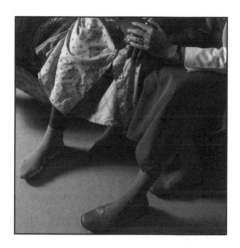

Sacred Time

I'm an RN. I always say that because I graduated from a hospital-based diploma school and I'm very proud of that. I have a BSN and a master's degree, and I'm also a Certified Hospice Palliative Nurse.

I work at an amazing place. Wishard Hospital is the inner city hospital for Indianapolis. It's a very creative institution—not a lot of money, but a lot of heart. I've been there 25 years and have worked in a variety of areas. For nearly 10 years I've been part of a team working on a large grant from the Soros Foundation, studying the dying poor.

We have interviewed patients who were terminally ill, along with their families, their caregivers, nurses, and doctors, and we asked them, "Tell us what it's like to be poor and dying." We sat in on focus groups and were amazed by their strength. So many people live emergency-room-visit to emergency-room-visit. We found that these patients were coming to the hospital and were being diagnosed with horrible illnesses, and then they'd say to us, "This is just the fifth bad thing that's happened to me this year."

We found out in the focus groups exactly what we thought we'd find: dying is dying, and it's hard for everyone. But it's especially hard for the poor, mainly because they can't tap into the resources that are available to the rest of us.

I'll make an assumption—if you or I were given a diagnosis of cancer, I know that at first I would be shocked and overwhelmed. I would experience the same feelings that everyone has when they are first confronted with this news. But, I know myself well enough to know that I would stay that way for a little while, but then I would move into action. I'd start thinking, "Who do I know? Who knows someone who knows about this condition? Who can I call?" I would start getting my support system really stirred up around me. I would be sending out messages that we need to form a prayer team. I know that I would get mobilized. The end result for everyone will be exactly the same, but I think you and I have the capability of tapping into more resources.

Can you tell me about someone you've recently worked with who falls into this category? How are these patients different from other patients we encounter?

Here's the difference with our patients. I have a patient who was diagnosed last week with metastatic liver cancer. It's bad, it's really bad. He had been feeling poorly and he knew something was wrong but didn't know what. This man is overwhelmed, he doesn't have health insurance, he doesn't have a 24/7 caregiver, and he doesn't feel well. And now he has to go home and manage all this, plus the emotions.

We're trying to stand in the gap with these patients and say, "Okay, we're recognizing this is a terrible situation. What can we do to help you? How can we help you manage this? And don't worry, because we're going to stick with you until the end. And, we'll stick with your family even beyond that."

There are 5 members on our team and we all work on the premise that we are given a wonderful opportunity every day to fall in love. We fall in love with these patients and thankfully we don't all fall in love with the same intensity. So we're not all going to be devastated by every patient we meet because some of us are more drawn to some patients than others. So we say, "We're going to partner with you. We'll help you find resources and help you have a better dying experience." I believe that people can die well.

There are 2 great privileges in nursing. The first is seeing babies born. It makes me believe that God wants us to go on. And the second is helping patients as they move through the dying process. Both situations are so much alike because in both instances patients are so vulnerable. It's such a sacred time in their lives and I'm honored to be part of that.

I'm often asked to speak on working with dying patients. There are a lot of groups that are interested in dying because we're all going to do it. So, I developed a list of the valuable life lessons that patients have taught me.

The first lesson is that there are worse things than dying. Physical, mental, and spiritual sufferings are just a few of those. I've also learned that patients give me so much more than I give them. I can't think of a single patient who hasn't taught me something about tenacity or hope, or spirituality. They are amazing teachers.

I've found that it's all about relationships, not possessions. Our dying patients form relationships with us very quickly. An initial consult with our team takes about an hour, and in that time we connect very quickly with them on a very intimate level. So, I have come to realize the importance of that connectiveness. I've learned that God has increased my capacity and ability to love even though my mortal sadness gets hooked when my patients die. I've learned that I'm blessed to be able to do my ministry at work, something that I believe God has called me to do.

There is something great and wonderful and fragile about every person. We take care of a variety of people here, including prisoners, and I still find it to be true. You make a difference in this world one person at a time. I've also learned that you live like you die, which makes me very aware of how I live my life. I've accepted the fact that I might not matter to a lot of people, but I matter a lot to a few people— and that has made me a better person.

I'd like to go back to something you said which really struck me. You said that your mortal sadness gets hooked, but that you are still able to go on doing the same work. Can you think of an experience with a patient where that was true?

I remember an absolutely delightful gentleman. We were originally taking care of his wife and I connected with him very quickly. He was such a nice man who obviously loved his wife a great deal and was extremely attentive to her as she was dying.

Not too long ago he called me and said, "You know Jo, I've got cancer and it's really bad." I told him I was sorry, and he continued, "Well you know, you did such a wonderful job helping me with my wife, I was wondering if you could help me." I asked him what it was that he thought I could do for him and he replied, "Oh, I'm not really expecting a whole lot. I'm just hoping you'll let me call you, or you'll call me, and that you'll get me connected with some resources. I just wanted you to know that."

I told him that I would be honored to help him. He called me several times. His pain medicine was making him miserable and he was having so much trouble with constipation. I had called his primary care physician and she was out of town but one of her partners was going to see him.

I went to the clinic just to be there with him and he said, "I know you're busy. Why did you come here?" I told him, "Because you're you and I enjoy being around you." I also wanted to talk to the doctor about trying a better pain regimen. It worked out so well.

After that, he called me when his granddaughter was born. They named her after him and he wanted me to know that. Then he called and told me he was coming to the hospital to have his feeding tube changed and he was hoping that I would see him. He said, "Your smile is worth so much to me." And I sat with him during part of the procedure.

We had a death in our family this past Christmas, and he died over Christmas as well. I remember our last meeting, looking at his face and thinking, "Ah—you know," and being sad because he was a lovely man. I just loved him, but now he's in heaven with his wife. It's that kind of sadness that we tap into.

You're working in an emotionally intense environment. How do you replenish yourself and make sure you're healthy enough to work with patients in this capacity?

I'm an early morning walker. I get up at 4:30 AM and I'm out walking before I go to work. I use that time to connect with God. It's a beautiful time of day, and I can be outside and be replenished looking at the sky and stars, thinking about how I am really just an infinitesimal speck and there is something much greater than me out there.

I'm very blessed that I'm part of a team and, fortunately for me, our chaplain is absolutely wonderful. We both look for meaning in things and she keeps me very aware that I need to be looking. I need to be able to name my feelings and work through those issues. We process a lot as a group, especially our difficult cases, so we get the opportunity to talk about feeling overwhelmed, wanting to cry, and talking about the unfairness in what we see. We're allowed to say those things out loud, and our feelings are validated.

Many times nurses don't have the opportunity to process their experiences as a group.

Exactly. We try to process with our nurses at Wishard. So many times they have invested a great deal in taking care of a dying patient and the patient is transferred to a nursing home or goes home. I always try to go back to the hospital nurse when I know of a death. I usually mention their obituary and show them the patient's picture. I always let them know they did a good job and were appreciated.

I don't remember dealing with so many deaths as a young nurse, but I do know that I've always been very close to my patients—sometimes in ways that probably weren't very good. I remember a gentleman I had taken care of in the emergency room who was a cardiac patient. He was always in and out of the hospital. One day he came in and looked worse than he had ever looked. I was hooking him up to the monitor and he went into ventricular fibrillation. I called the code, started the IV, and called the doctor. We worked and worked, but in the end we lost him. I remember the doctor looking at me and saying, "We'll call the code now. It's done." But

I couldn't accept that. I told him, "You cannot do that. We have to try again."

It was so difficult for me because I had seen him pull out of so many situations in the past. The doctor actually excused me out of the room and said, "I need you to leave. I need you to get yourself a drink of water or a pop, but I need you out of this room." I told him I wasn't sure that I could leave, but he was very kind and said he'd find someone to help me. Eventually I did leave, and he talked with me and processed what we experienced. And then he did something absolutely wonderful. He looked at me and said, "I'd like you to go with me when we talk to his daughter. You cared about him so much, and I think she would want to know that."

You're doing amazing work. I'm sure your patients and families appreciate you.

It's easier for some families than others to tell you that, but for the most part we know that what we do makes a difference, and that makes doing the hard stuff easier.

I remember one patient very distinctly because I was still a fairly young nurse working in the ICU. A father had backed his car over his 2-year-old daughter. Can you imagine? I had a 2-year-old child at the time and I remember calling the babysitter and saying, "I know Ryan is asleep, but I just need to know that he's okay."

The father of that poor little girl just wanted to be in the room with her, and all I could say was that this was very difficult and we weren't expecting her to live. It was heart-wrenching. Holding back the tears, he responded, "I caused it. I have to be here." I remember the two of us holding hands and watching her die. I also went to the funeral.

Do you think these experiences were turning points for you? In some way they were preparing you for the work you're currently doing?

I hadn't thought about it that way, but that does make sense.

I'm getting fairly close to retiring, so I think a lot about selecting the right person to take my place. I think a lot about how you choose this person, and what makes people interested in palliative care. I don't know what allowed me to think that I could do this.

And when you do find that person who will take over your work, what do you think his or her qualities should be?

I want them to recognize that it's a privilege to sit with patients at a time when they are extremely vulnerable. Those patients need your respect in order to be vulnerable with you. I would ask their intentions in applying for this position. Is it because I wear regular clothes instead of scrubs? Is it because you see I don't work nights and weekends? If I don't hear that they want this job because they want to help people who are in the process of dying, then I'm inclined to believe it's not something they really want to do. There is nothing glamorous about this work. You don't have the adrenaline rush you have in the Emergency Department, and it's not the ICU, but some of my greatest moments have come when I'm sitting at a patient's bedside doing absolutely nothing but holding his or her hand and praying.

How did you choose nursing?

I'm a highly caring person and I think I was probably drawn to medicine because of my grandmother. She was a nursing assistant at our local hospital and I always loved hearing about the patients she worked with and the interesting things she did. So I became a nursing assistant in high school and worked summers in preparation for college. I actually thought about being a physician, but I had a guidance counselor who told me that I wasn't bright enough. I graduated tenth in my class, but that was 1967 and women didn't pursue those types of careers. Today I understand what a terrible thing that was for someone to say.

So, I decided to become a nurse and entered a baccalaureate program. The university was far from home and overall I didn't think it was the right program for me. I had been a nursing assistant for several summers, and back then nursing assistants did a lot. Here I was in a baccalaureate program, a very good program, and I wasn't even going to have a nursing class until the first semester of my second year. I was just unhappy. So, I left the university but found that there was a diploma program close to my hometown. I applied for it and was accepted. In a diploma program, you practice nursing right away. I thought, "This is it!" I am so grateful for that kind of basic training because I feel that it allowed me to be a hands-on nurse first. Do I wish now I understood a little more clearly that it's very difficult to advance up the ranks with just a diploma? Of course, but I've had some very neat experiences because I did it exactly the way I did it.

Looking to the future, how can we strengthen our profession?

There are so many nurses in this country but we're not active in the political arena. Who understands health care better than a nurse? I mean the nuts and bolts of health care. No one. We're so integral in making that process work. I don't know what has caused us to feel like we don't need to be politically active or we shouldn't be involved.

Our problem today is a shortage of faculty, and the reason is low pay. Nurses at the bedside earn more than faculty, and nurses in the hospital setting earn more than nurses in the community. How can we bring more nurses into the profession when there is such a disparity in salaries?

The issue always comes back to money. By the way, we never talked about how your program is funded. In addition to the grant from the Soros Foundation, how does this program stay solvent?

Less than 40% of our patients are insured, so the hospital covers the remaining cost. And do you know why they do it? Because it's the right thing to do. Our program will never make money. If we break even we'll consider ourselves lucky. But it is the right thing to do, and it makes a difference in people's lives. These patients have limited resources, and dying is hard. We can make that process easier for them. They deserve it.

Jo, do you consider your work to be heroic?

Heroic? When I think of heroes I certainly don't think of myself. I know that there are people who look at me and might think that I am, but do I think it? No. I think I'm fortunate. My patients are amazing, and I stand in awe of them every day. I've been given an amazing opportunity to do this work.

Jo A. Groves, RN, MS, CHPN
Clinical Nurse Palliative Care
Indiana

CHAPTER 28

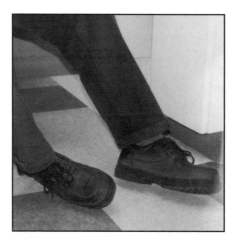

Rebel With a Cause

I started as a nursing assistant in a nursing home when I was 14 years old. I loved it. I loved caring for geriatric patients, and I worked with friends and mentors who taught me the meaning of good patient care. When I was 16, I filed a formal complaint with the Department of Public Health because the quality of patient care at the nursing home had dropped significantly, and I witnessed patient abuse.

I was fired a week later.

I realized that as an aide, I had no power or authority to change that situation. The only way I could have made a significant impact was if I had been a nurse. Seven years later, I was a registered nurse working for an agency at the height of the nursing shortage in the late 1980s. Agency nursing meant carrying a heavy patient assignment on under-staffed units.

I remember taking care of a young man diagnosed with HIV-AIDS. We didn't know that much about it then, and there were people genuinely fearful of that diagnosis. He wasn't receiving the best care, and that made me furious. Although I was assigned to 15 other patients, I took the time to assess his pain and carefully clean his wounds. I guess that is what drives me—being an advocate for the underdog. I saw myself as someone who could protect them.

What would you say is the essence of nursing?

Selfless compassion. It is how well we care for our patients and ourselves. To be a good nurse, you need to be passionate about your work, but you also need a level of detachment. I also think that your intuitive sense as a nurse is your biggest asset.

Would you consider any of your patient interactions to be heroic?

When you read about it in the third person they could be, but I didn't go into nursing expecting rewards. Recognition comes in small, simple ways: a smile from a patient, or how a family member looks at you.

Any final thoughts?

We need to share more as nurses. We need better outlets and support for the work we do.

Thomas P. Koppes, BSN, RN
Clinical Research Coordinator
Illinois

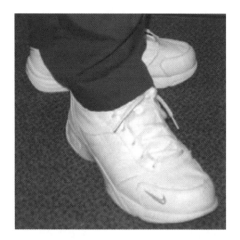

CHAPTER 29

The Courage to Advocate

I have been a nurse at Waukesha Memorial Hospital for 6 years. This is where I want to work. As a child I remember being interested in hospitals but in high school I didn't think I'd qualify to go into nursing. Several years ago my nephew was rushed to this hospital where he died of SIDS (Sudden Infant Death Syndrome). Everyone was so wonderful and caring, and I was so impressed by the way they treated our whole family. I have never had a bad experience here, and I knew that I wanted to be a part of that.

Shortly after that experience I started working as a nursing assistant in long-term care, and all of the nurses I worked with encouraged me to follow my dream and become an RN. I wish I could go back there and thank them all for their support. I just needed a little push.

I work with patients who have a variety of diagnoses, and I learn something new every day. We see patients with pneumonia, chronic obstructive pulmonary disease, cellulitis, pressure ulcers, stroke, and cardiac disease. I've also worked with a patient who had Desert Fever. You learn the basics in school, but there is still a lot of learning to be done on a daily basis. It takes a special kind of nurse to work on this unit, someone who has the common sense to work through patient problems and not take things personally. You also need to follow your gut feeling.

Have you always had that gut feeling?

Yes, although I didn't listen to it in the beginning. A lot of it was self-doubt, being a new nurse. Now I know that I have to act on it every time. It's almost like a premonition, or a nagging feeling that won't go away until you address it. I've worked with enough patients that I can tell if something is not right with them. It comes from experience.

There was a young woman several years ago who had a severe lung infection and had to have her lung removed. We had to be strong advocates for this patient because we wanted her to get better, and we needed the whole team to work together. She was on a ventilator and couldn't speak, so we learned to read her lips in order to communicate. She became close to a lot of us. Eventually she got better, was able to attend rehab, and eventually she went home.

She was employed at a local department store where I was shopping one day and I saw that she was on duty. It was the most wonderful feeling to see her looking so well. I got such a thrill from that.

She recognized me and came over and said, "I just wanted to thank you for all you did. Please say hello to everyone for me." Now she'll visit the unit every once in a while and bring treats for everyone. She went through so much and still had a positive attitude toward us! It made me feel good to know that we were doing the right things for her in the hospital.

What did you learn from that experience?

I learned not to get discouraged because sometimes things do take longer than usual. I also learned that I should never be afraid to be a patient advocate. I would want someone to advocate for me if I were in that situation.

Would you consider your actions to be heroic?

As nurses we often don't give ourselves enough credit. There have been times when we've saved lives, and some days we go above and beyond. I'd call that heroic.

Carol Majeskie, RN
Charge Nurse, Medical Surgical Department
Wisconsin

CHAPTER 30

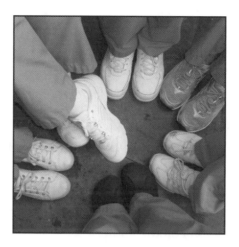

A Walk Down the Aisle

I have worked in the information technology industry for 30 years, and now I am in nursing school. The interesting thing is, I'm not the oldest person in my cohort. We range in age from 19 to 52 years.

What made you choose nursing as a second career?

I always wanted to be a nurse. I was a candy striper when I was a teenager, and I've done a lot of volunteer work and been involved in various humanitarian efforts over the years. My daughter is grown and my stepdaughter is in college; I had the opportunity to go back to school, so I did.

We're experiencing a nursing faculty shortage which is impacting the admission process. Did you apply to very many programs?

I applied to 10 different schools and all of them were in California. Some were associate degree programs, with a waiting list of more than 3 years, and there were a few baccalaureate programs that relied on a point system for admission. I'm in a brand new baccalaureate program at California State University San Marcos and I'll be in the first cohort to be graduating next May. The program consists of 8 semesters taken over the course of 3 years, once you've completed your prerequisite classes.

Is it what you expected it to be?

Pretty much. I didn't think it was going to be easy. My sister is a telemetry nurse, so I knew it was going to be a challenge. I didn't expect a walk in the park.

What made you choose this school?

I took a bioethics class that was taught by the dean of the nursing school, and I was so impressed with her demeanor and her whole way of thinking that I decided her program was the right one for me. She really stretched you to not only look at your morals, but at other points of view and taking a whole cultural look at ethics. We have a wide range of cultures in California. Not only are there large Hispanic and Asian populations here, but we have a growing Russian and Ukrainian population as well.

I love nursing school and I love being with patients. I'm on a telemetry unit now and I'm assigned 4 patients. I started with 1 patient, but as I learned the unit and became more comfortable, they gradually increased my assignment to four. With 4 patients you really have to learn time management skills.

It helps that our school offers an internship program, which is an unpaid work experience where they pair you with a preceptor for 96 to 108 hours and have you manage a patient assignment.

This semester we have an opportunity to do an externship, which is a paid position. It is similar to the internship, but with slightly more responsibility.

How was it working with the nurses on the units? Are they appreciative of student nurses or are there challenges there?

There have been some challenges. The internship that I did was very difficult, mainly as a result of the preceptor, but that has been my only negative experience so far. They offered to change preceptors, but I was nearly finished with the program, so I decided to stick it out. I look at that as a learning experience because you don't always get along with every coworker.

How does the school help you prepare for this type of assignment?

We have a great lab. We have 6 Smarties. I used to call them Dummies, but they're not. They're very high-tech manikins. We set up a hospital ward, similar to an emergency room, with 6 beds and 6 Smarties to practice with. You can actually insert nasogastric tubes and check blood pressures. We have one manikin that can accommodate chest tubes and can be programmed for a code situation. The best part is whenever we work with the manikins, we are videotaped so that we can watch and critique our skills.

I told my simulation lab instructor about an experience I had with a nurse educator on the unit. I was assigned a patient who had a chest tube, and when the nurse educator asked me questions about chest tubes, I was able to answer all of them because of my experience in the lab. I knew about looping, and what to look for in the bubbling because we had done a simulation in the lab.

The simulations are very real. When we set up a patient code in the lab, my heart was racing because I couldn't find a pulse and I thought my patient was going to die. We made mistakes, but it's better to make mistakes there so we can learn from them. In that patient code situation someone forgot to insert the backboard before starting CPR, and we learned from experience that you can't do CPR in a soft bed. I know none of us will ever do that again.

The manikins can be programmed to interact with you, which makes it even more real. The instructor is actually in the next room behind a one-way mirror and programs the manikin to say it doesn't feel well, or is nauseated, etc. Sometimes the instructor will give you little hints when you're having a hard time figuring out what to do next.

The other thing I love about the simulation lab is that it's a true learning experience. We're not graded on our work with the manikins. Instead, we're graded on our care plans. People make tons of mistakes in there, but you learn from that.

From your 30 years of experience in IT, tell me what you think about the hospital's use of technology and what you think might be areas for improvement.

Well, I think that hospitals are way behind the times, technologically. There is a national health care system that promotes computer charting, but it's a DOS-based program and, despite its claims, the nurses are still hand charting their assessments. That is probably because the program is not very user friendly. People are more familiar with Windows based applications.

I've also worked on units that have several computers on wheels (COWs) that are portable, wireless laptops that nurses can wheel around from room to room. Half of them don't work, and other times the wireless system is down. Nurses are expected to chart everything exactly, and that's difficult to do when you're searching for the only COW on the unit that is working.

I agree with you, and feel that we need to take a closer look at our work environment and make sure that at the very least, the equipment works.

I think they should have a computer in every patient room. This way the patient is exposed to one less potential contaminant.

I don't want to criticize, but because of my background, I notice the glitches.

Have you thought about where you'd like to work after graduation?

My first goal is to graduate before I have to walk down the aisle with a walker! (laughter) I really thought that I would work in women's health, but the longer I am in school, the more I think I need to wait before making a decision. I like the ICU, but I'd also like to try community health. I had the opportunity to shadow a TB nurse and found that I enjoyed seeing people in their homes. It's a totally different kind of nursing. It's not so much technology as it is working one-on-one with people.

I'd like to ask you a question based on the title of this book. Do you consider any of your actions as a student nurse to be heroic?

I think it depends on your definition of heroic. I've never saved anyone's life, but I feel like I've made a difference in somebody's life. It might have been a tiny, tiny difference but that's my goal. Every day when I go to the hospital I try to make that person's life just a tiny bit better.

Mary Baker
Student Nurse
California

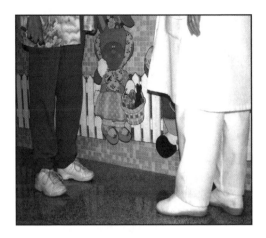

Raising the Bar

I grew up in a family where you were either a nurse or a nun, or both. As a form of rebellion, I decided to be neither, but that was short-lived. Nursing won, and I have been a nurse for nearly 40 years.

My mom grew up during the Depression. She wanted to be a nurse, but couldn't afford to go to nursing school. On my father's side, I'd say that about 25 out of 30 females were nurses. Initially, I wanted to be a history teacher, but after my first year in college, I decided to switch to nursing. I saw so many history teachers out of work because there weren't enough jobs. I also realized that I could make a real difference as a nurse.

Have you succeeded in making a difference?

Oh yes. I look back and remember how many teams I've built, and lost, and built again. To think of those nurses I trained who are now in other specialties....they got their med-surg experience from me, and I think they became better, more well-rounded nurses as a result.

How would you differentiate your med-surg nurses from other specialties?

I mean this in the most complimentary way: my med-surg nurses are the workhorses in this hospital. They're not afraid to work, they're not afraid of hard labor. These nurses are good people. I'd like to think that I raised them to be that way.

Medical-surgical nursing is a specialty. These patients are so complex and have so many co-morbidities. There is constant change. I'm still excited about my job. I'm still learning.

You've been a manager for more than 30 years. Is there a secret to your success?

I've always said that what I want written on my tombstone is that I was fair. Some nurses might say that I'm tough, but it's really that I set my expectations high—but not unreasonably so. You don't expect a nurse to call-in lightly.

Right now I'm dealing with the unique situation of working with several generations on the same unit. I have 4 generations working with me: the Veterans, Baby Boomers, Generation X-ers and the Next-ers, and you need to find out what motivates each group. My role is to groom people to improve.

Would you consider any of your actions or interventions as a nurse to be heroic?

Absolutely. I consider myself to be a risk taker. I've always spoken up for nurses and for patients throughout my career.

Marguerite Svenson, RN, MS
Director, Medical Patient Care
Illinois

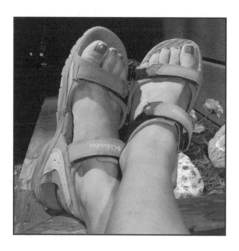

CHAPTER 32

Universal Caregiver

When people say, "Oh, you're a nurse!" the next question should be, "What do you do?" because that could be anything.

You are a good case in point. You've worked in oncology, home health and hospice, critical care, and now you are a Family Nurse Practitioner. You are even a camp nurse for your children. And to top it all off, you are a Major in the US Air Force Reserves, Nurse Corps. Did you know from a very young age that you'd like to be a nurse?

I don't remember growing up saying I wanted to be a nurse. As a matter of fact, my mother was quite surprised when I told her years later. She told me I always hated the sight of blood! I just knew I wanted to help people in general, and it got funneled into joining the military and then the medical field. The nurses I met in the military were such amazing people and that's when I thought that maybe I could do this.

It still amazes me how quickly and easily you can form relationships with people on a very intimate level, which is something you could never do being their accountant.

When I first graduated, I had no idea in what area of nursing I wanted to work. The nurse recruiter told me that the oncology unit always seemed calm and asked if I wanted to take a tour. All of the nurses had a very special way about them and seemed accepting. I liked the unit and took the job.

This was in Hawaii in 1991. I moved there from Massachusetts, where they had a nursing surplus and my friends from school could only find jobs as Certified Nursing Assistants (CNAs) in nursing homes. For 10 years I worked in oncology, then home health and hospice.

Being a hospice nurse made an impression on me. It's such an honor having people wanting me to be with them as they die. I remember working as a hospice nurse with 2 elderly sisters. They were widowed and now were living together. I was seeing the sister with dementia regularly, and I quickly became part of the family. My patient had passed away early in the morning and her sister called me. I was the first person she called, even before her own daughter.

I'll never forget that call. "Monsita," she said, "I'd just like you to come here and be with me." I was so honored that I was the first person she thought of.

I was in the military in the nurse corps at the same time, which focused on trauma training, and I felt like I was trying to practice 2 specialties at different ends of the spectrum. That was difficult for me so I decided to change my civilian job to critical care nursing. I still work per diem in critical care, and now I'm a flight nurse in the Reserves.

Have you traveled to many conflict areas?

I've been on missions where we flew to Afghanistan, picked up patients and brought them back to Ramstein Air Base, where I was stationed in Germany. The patients then transferred to nearby Landstuhl Army Hospital. We'd rest for a day or so and go on another mission, this time to Iraq. From Germany, the patients were eventually transported to Washington, DC.

How safe do you feel traveling to these areas of the world?

I feel very safe. Mainly because our aircraft are very expensive commodities and the pilots are highly trained. There hasn't been a flight carrying patients in a large cargo aircraft that has gone down since the Vietnam War.

We transport between 12 and 70 patients per mission. The aircraft is a C-17 (the C stands for cargo), and we set it up like an ICU. We arrange our stations and equipment, and set up the electrical and oxygen outlets. Setting up the aircraft is demanding, physical work, and then we turn around and start caring for the patients! That's the real work.

The nursing care is the same kind of care we provide in the hospital, but at a higher altitude. In Ramstein you get a preliminary report and when you land, the report changes [laughs]. They're always trying to add more patients at the last minute. But you're there for the soldiers. They're such heroes and I'm proud to be part of a team that's bringing them home. That's a bonus for me.

Is there a particular mission that stands out for you?

There is. It has to do with a little boy, and I can't remember if this was Iraq or Afghanistan. When you fly into a foreign country in the middle of the night, your main concern is caring for your patient, not in which country you're landing.

This little boy suffered severe burns as a result of a propane tank explosion. He was accompanied by his mother, who spoke very little English. She sat next to me and the military interpreter, and we struck up a conversation. She showed me pictures of her son before the accident and I could tell she was so proud of him. I told her he was a beautiful little boy; tears filled her eyes and she began to cry.

What surprised me is that the interpreter told me she thought I was wonderful. But I hadn't done anything! I wasn't even her son's nurse. We were just talking about our lives and our children. I had told her about being a nurse in the military, and we shared our stories. We were two women sitting side-by-side, but coming from very different worlds. I was in my military uniform and she was wearing a burka, with perfectly matching black purse and shoes. I wondered what she was thinking, and at the same time I was incredibly appreciative of how I grew up and of all of the opportunities afforded to me.

That was a powerful, singular experience for me, but I'm also moved by seeing the young men and women, barely 18 years old, coming back home after having suffered a head injury or missing a limb. I'm a mom and I don't know how I'd feel about my own children in that position. Being a nurse in the military is such a neat thing because we're not the aggressors. We're there to help whomever; it doesn't matter. I just know that my contribution is helping.

You're a universal caregiver. You've practiced nursing in different parts of this country and the world, working with a variety of cultures. In addition to your military service, you're also a Family Practice Nurse Practitioner. Where are you working?

I work in a community clinic where we see a lot of homeless people and migrant workers. Sadly, the majority of our patients don't have health insurance. I love this work, but there are challenges. I thought I'd have enough time to fully explore the possibilities of a diagnosis and I'm finding that we're just not given enough time to do that effectively.

Are you compensated adequately for your work as a Nurse Practitioner?

Oh no [laughs]. I chose to work in a community health clinic, and they're one of the lowest payers, but I had no idea that I would be earning only $4 more per hour as a Nurse Practitioner than as a critical care nurse working per diem in a hospital. This is sad, because I still have to pay for my professional liability insurance and continuing education credits, etc. Once you add up all the expenses, I'm probably making less than in my critical care position. I don't think that people in the community know that we're not being compensated adequately.

I understand the Doctorate of Nursing Practice (DNP) will become the new entry level into practice for Nurse Practitioners. Do you have any thoughts on that?

I can make the argument for both sides. On one hand I wonder, "What are they thinking?" We're not even being compensated at the master's level, and now we're asking people to go for their DNP and take on more debt for the same pay scale?

A major selling point for introducing Nurse Practitioners as one solution to the health care crisis is the fact that NPs don't cost as much. But if you're going to mandate having a DNP, NPs will be asking for greater compensation, which will reduce that difference.

On the other hand, I've always been a big proponent of education. I roll my eyes whenever I hear the arguments comparing the ADN nurse and the BSN (I entered the profession as an ADN nurse), because I look at the bigger picture, and I see what the public sees: every other ancillary service in health care has a graduate degree for entry into practice, except nursing. Every other service didn't have a 20 year-long debate on whether we should increase the education level. They just did it. They knew health care was becoming so complex and dynamic that they needed someone educated at a higher level.

I'm frustrated and passionate about this because I understand both sides of the doctorate issue. There are strong points made in favor of pursuing higher education for this level of practitioner, but in the real world, how can you tell someone, "We'll pay you $37 per hour, but you'll have to get your doctorate first."

That's why I don't completely hate it that we're moving so fast on the DNP. I'm impressed that things are moving along so quickly. But as usual are we going in the right direction?

As I said, I love my work, and I enjoy the patients I work with. I'm very happy to be a Nurse Practitioner, in spite of the challenges. I'm especially happy that as an NP I no longer need to use nursing diagnoses. We use medical diagnoses instead. I could never understand why they were created in the first place. I don't believe it really helped the patient when we wrote, "Alteration in comfort related to…" when, in fact, the patient was in pain.

There was discussion and debate years ago about defining nursing as a profession, and as such, needing its own language. And so, nursing diagnoses came into being. Was the reason for bettering patient care, or for professional self-promotion? We could have more long discussions about students using nursing diagnoses to help develop critical thinking skills, but we should always evaluate any change in practice by asking ourselves, "Will this improve patient care?"

You've had so many interesting experiences and have touched so many lives, would you consider your work as a nurse to be heroic?

I'd have a hard time saying that about myself. When I think of heroic, I think of putting myself in either physical danger or moral danger; an ethical dilemma. I'm not sure I've ever had to do that. I've had patient care conferences where I've had to stand up to a physician and press a little harder for issues I thought were important for the patient, but hadn't been identified. We've had different points of view, but I don't think that's heroic. And I've never felt personally in danger on any of my missions.

I just try to put my patients first. Take for instance, the soldiers we AirEvac from the Middle East to Germany and on to the United States. They can be traveling up to 3 to 4 days sometimes. That's an awfully long time to be traveling even if you're well, so you can imagine what it feels like to be a patient in that situation.

On one of my last missions I gave my patient a bed bath—well, more like a head-to-toe clean up. All I could think of was how badly this guy needed a bath. Think about it. The nurses in Baghdad or Afghanistan are dealing with traumas. They're doing everything possible to save a life, and then they bundle up the patient for the long flight home. So I thought, 'I've got a long flight ahead of me and I'm not doing anything else, I'm going to clean this guy up.'

I felt so much better afterward. He didn't like it in the beginning because he didn't want to move. Even though I medicated him for pain, it never seems like it's enough. I had to insist, "I really have to do this." Afterward he mouthed, "Thank you," and I thought, "Yeah. That's my gold star."

You know, the little things in nursing like that aren't heroic. It's just something that I would want someone to do for me.

Monsita Foley, RN, MSN, FNP-BC
Major, US Air Force Reserve, Nurse Corps
California

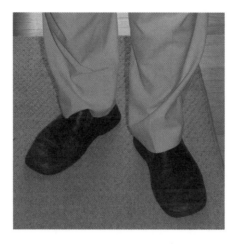

CHAPTER 33

Nice to Meet You

Every time I think I'm getting burned out in nursing, something always happens to rejuvenate me.

I am a psychiatric nurse and not too long ago, when I thought I was losing that spark, I began working with a man who was diagnosed with catatonic schizophrenia. He was so ill that he couldn't even feed himself. To make matters worse, he reverted back to his primary language, which is Spanish.

I was able to work with him one-on-one and I tried my best to communicate with him in Spanish. I used phrase books and dictionaries to remind him that he needed to eat and take his medications. The communication barrier was very frustrating for me, but as he got better, his English also improved. It took nearly a week, but he finally addressed me and said, "Nice to meet you. My name is Jim."

I couldn't believe it. I was happy and relieved at the same time. I looked at him and said, "Nice to meet you, my ass! I've been working with you for 7 days!" We both laughed! It was so rewarding to see him making progress. His memory was still very cloudy, which was a good thing because he was very tormented during that time.

It's times like these that remind me why I became a nurse.

Do you consider any of your interventions at work to be heroic?

Actually, when I was doing the initial assessment on a patient a while back, I had a sense that something was wrong. This wasn't a typical psychosis or depression. When I called the doctor with my assessment later that evening I told him my concerns and added, "I think there is something unusual going on here. Can we get a CT scan of his head?"

The next morning one of the nurses called me at home and congratulated me. When I asked her why, she said, "Your patient had his CT scan and they found a neoplasm in his brain the size of a medium orange! He was rushed to surgery and had it removed."

Here's the best part. The insurance company rep called the physician and demanded, "What was your justification for ordering a CT scan of the brain for a patient on a psych floor?" The doctor calmly responded, "Well, the patient had a rather large neoplasm in the brain." "And how did you pick that up?" asked the rep.

Without missing a beat, the doctor replied, "I didn't. The nurse did."

Ed Shilney, RN, BSN
Registered Hypnotherapist
Staff Nurse, Psychiatric and Substance Abuse
Illinois

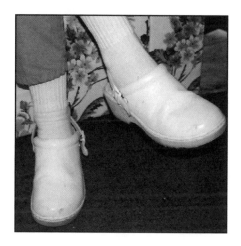

CHAPTER 34

I See Miracles Every Day

When I was in college I wanted to be a dietitian. I really believe that what you eat affects your health. However, the school I was in didn't offer a degree in nutrition, so I chose nursing.

I love babies and new mothers and new life—I just thrive on that. I can't teach the moms enough and I can't look at babies enough. I'll never get over looking babies and seeing how beautiful and perfect they are. After 15 years, I'm still excited about going to work!

I've always worked with moms and babies, and now I'm a lactation consultant as well. In addition to my work at the hospital, I have an online business selling breast pumps and breastfeeding accessories. I also make home visits to see new mothers.

Is there a particular experience in your career that stands out?

There are so many! I'm especially moved by adoption situations. People think that those babies aren't loved at all, but I've been with those moms and I can tell you that is absolutely not true. It's the most precious love I've ever seen in my life. I saw a 17 year old kiss every millimeter of her baby before giving her up. She loved that baby enough to know that she just couldn't keep her, and was noble enough to allow another couple to adopt her child.

I told that story several years ago to a young girl at a party. Wouldn't you know it, 6 months later she became pregnant. She wrote to me to say that the relationship fell apart even before the baby was born, and that she was going to give the baby up for adoption because of my story. It was such a difficult decision for her to make and she knew that I wouldn't judge her.

Would you consider your work to be heroic?

Of course! I can't tell you the number of times I've done CPR on a baby. I've saved lives.

Noreen Shilney, RN, BSN, IBCLC
Lactation Consultant
Illinois

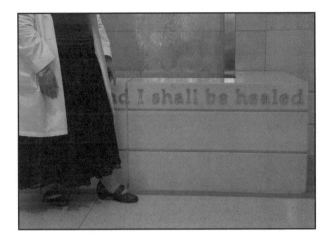

CHAPTER 35

Open Heart

"Place me where you need me to be."

That was my prayer for months before I was offered my current position as the Clinical Resource Nurse for cardiovascular services. I didn't want to take just any job and find out later it wasn't right. I've been a nurse for 24 years and there are places where I knew I couldn't work. I don't share the same philosophy of nursing with some hospitals. They might look beautiful on the outside, but being in those environments does not feed your spirit.

Before I had my first interview for this job I came to the hospital just to see how I would feel in this environment. It was a brand new hospital section and still a hard-hat area, and the first thing I noticed was the water wall. It wasn't running yet, but I saw the inscription at the base which read, "Only say the word and I shall be healed." That's my absolute favorite part of the Catholic mass, and I knew at that moment that this was the right fit for me.

And so here I am at this new place doing exactly what I love to do, mentoring and teaching, spending lots of time with patients and families and helping set a new tone in this new hospital with a new model of care. And it gets better. I recently got a call—from out of the blue—from one of the administrators asking if I'd be interested in joining their team exploring the palliative care process within an acute care setting. This is precisely what I'd like to focus on in my doctoral degree. I accepted the invitation and offered them a name for the project: Mors Bella, which is Latin for beautiful death. We chose Bella Morte, a term that is often encountered within end-of-life literature.

I've always been interested in thanatology, which is the study of death and dying. I find it fascinating, not frightening at all. I had the privilege of midwifing my mother's own death, which helped me realize what a beautiful moment it can be. Very early in my career I discovered I had a capacity for listening, and when a patient really needed to pass on I was often the one who could open up that conversation and guide the patient and family through the process. It became the focus of my master's work: critical care nurses' perceptions of patient advocacy during end of life care. I wanted to know if it was a sensitivity borne out of being an experienced and expert nurse in the Benner tradition or was it borne out of life experience, no matter what stage of nursing the professional found him- or herself in.

Would you share a situation in which you helped a patient or his family through this process?

When I worked in critical care, there were times when patients were comatose at my first encounter with them, but there existed a family dynamic at the bedside from which I could determine who this man or woman was lying in that bed. I could tell who needed what kind of healing in order to release this person by listening very closely.

There are times when people will sacrifice themselves for the sake of a loved one. The fact of their illness or of their death will alter the course of the lives around them. My mother spent the last 9 years of her life in a coma, and there were so many times when she was a whisper away from dying. She would somehow pull through repeated sepsis crises, against all odds, over the 9 years. I know that she stayed on this side until I could "afford" to let her go. I had a year as a professional nurse, well-established in my independence. It was in the moment of her death that I realized the whole language of her illness. And so it is with many patients and their families. I look at the family situation and try to understand what is going on, and I really listen to how each person relates to that patient in the bed.

I remember one family where 2 brothers would not speak to each other because 1 brother had married outside the faith. Whenever Michael would walk into his father's room the other would walk out. Thank goodness there was a peacemaker in the family. Dan was the neutral brother of the 5 children. The brothers would continue to visit, but it was always a tense situation when their paths crossed.

One afternoon I realized that their father was getting closer and closer to death. He was DNR ("do not resuscitate"), which would offer the family the chance to have an uninterrupted experience at the bedside for the end. When Dan came to visit alone, I explained to him about heart rhythms and what to look for on the monitor. I told him to look at the heart rhythm and see what type of pattern it was making on the screen. I asked him to imagine a weave in a sweater and if you had a string and started to pull, it would keep the shape of the original weave until you began pulling it further and further out....and eventually it would go straight.

"So what you're going to see," I told him, "is that little first bump called the P-wave. It's going to start moving away from the high part called the QRS. Eventually, the QRS is going to get pulled apart, getting wider and wider and eventually it's going to be just a little squiggle, and then it's going to be a flat line."

Dan looked at the monitor as I was talking and started to see the changes in his father's heart rhythm. "Am I starting to see what you're talking about?" he asked.

"Yes, you are. I need you to get your family." But he hesitated because Michael, the outcast brother, and his wife were also there. He looked at me and I said, "That's right, bring everyone."

Dan brought everyone into his father's room, and even though there was bristling and resentment, I stood there quietly and said, "I'm glad that you're here. It's important for all of you to be here right now." As I adjusted their father's IVs, I began humming "Amazing Grace" very softly. It's one of those songs that everyone knows and it transcends religions. Before I knew it, one of the sisters started humming and pretty soon every single person standing there was singing out loud. While this was happening, my patient's heart rate slowed and faltered, and he died peacefully with his entire family surrounding him. Everyone cried and embraced in that moment. I knew it was very important to the father to have that rift settled. There's more to heaven and earth than meets the eye.

Mors Bella....beautiful death. I think you've described it beautifully.

I also love working with heart patients; they are the best. They have a certain vulnerability, and there is something I have in common with them. I've also had a sternotomy, and when you've had that sternal bone breached, you realize just how vulnerable you are as a human being. There is nothing, nothing like having the protection of your heart compromised and feeling a click, click, click whenever you move, sneeze, bend forward, or turn to your side. Very little stands between me and my heart. It's an amazing feeling.

Patients don't like to talk about it because it's so frightening for them, but I've shared my story with a few patients to help ease their fear. I remember one patient who looked around the room nervously and whispered to me, "How soon before I feel human?"

"Wait until the first time you sneeze!" I laughed. "You'll be looking for your heart on the other side of the room! There's nothing you can do to stop it so just go with it." He wanted to know if the feeling of vulnerability goes away, and I reassured him that it does, but it'll take a while.

Health care is going through tremendous changes. Where do you see the future of our profession?

We have a young staff on our unit, and I told them that in 5 years I want them to be a team that is cohesive and strong, because let's face it, I'm likely to be their patient in another 4 or 5 years. I want them to be powerful diagnostically, powerful therapeutically, and powerful spiritually, to treat a person like myself who wants the same level of care that I would give to any one of them were our roles reversed.

I've noticed a trend recently that some young nurses push themselves into a master's program so quickly that they rush in with only 1 or 2 years of nursing experience under their belts. They start working toward becoming an advance practice nurse and I think they confuse having a master's in nursing with being a masterful nurse.

I also think we should have an almost evangelical spirit in terms of insisting that this next generation is qualified to serve on every level. We're graduating nurses right, left, and center who come out with enough general knowledge to pass the NCLEX exam but we have lost a lot of the humanizing elements having a generation largely raised without the humanities. How many students today have any sense of literature, philosophy, or the arts that teach us so much about the human spirit? We have lost much of that within American popular culture. It is time to pull ourselves back to the center as a nation.

I'd like to tell nurses just entering the field to slow down and really absorb the gestalt of nursing. As a novice nurse, you might be able to speak the language, but you don't have the naturalness of someone who is fluent. That takes time and years of practice. I'll sometimes ask a new nurse if he or she plays a musical instrument. Take the piano, for instance. Do you remember the first time you ever sat on the bench looking at the keys, then looking at the music and back again at the keys? How were you after your fourth year? You probably weren't even looking at the keys anymore. Nursing is a lot like that. As a new nurse you're going to be looking at every step in order to complete the tasks at hand. Performing the skills of nursing is going to take all of your energy. The art of nursing will come later.

You've mentioned both the art and the science of nursing. Would you consider your work as a nurse to be heroic?

Oh, absolutely! Both of my brothers are physicians and they have both said to me, "Nurses are really the heart of medicine, aren't they?"

I believe we truly are. You can be a proficient nurse in terms of getting the medication to the bedside in a timely manner and completing all of your charting, but when it comes to being a true healer, that's a different matter altogether. We give patients back their dignity in so many ways and we find that gentle moment to help them reconnect with themselves.

We give patients the courage to heal.

Karen Thomas, MS, RN
Clinical Resource Nurse
Cardiovascular Service Line
Illinois

SECTION FOUR

"We will be known forever by the tracks we leave."

Dakota Proverb

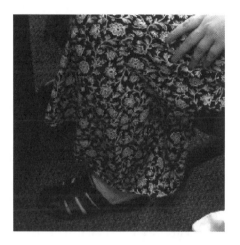

CHAPTER 36

Serendipity

Ioften tell my students a funny story about how I knew I would be
a good nurse. I always knew I'd be a nurse. That wasn't a big decision for me. I liked science and I liked working with people and
the rest just fell into place. A lot of students tell me they're inspired
by their mother or a relative who's in the profession, but while I had
an aunt who was a nurse, I wouldn't say that she inspired me. She just
helped put nursing on the radar for me.

My mother didn't think it was a good fit though, and told me that I
should consider volunteering as a candy striper so I'd have some idea
of what I was getting into. As a sophomore in high school I soon realized there was a hierarchy in candy striping. Everyone wanted to be
with the babies or deliver flowers, which created a 2-year wait in those
areas. The only places that would take you right away were the adult/
senior care areas. It didn't matter to me where I worked, so I accepted
an opening on an adult unit.

On my first day I was assigned to fill patients' water pitchers, and
the nurse gave me a list of all the patients who could have ice. This
was only 30 years ago, but it might as well have been the olden days

when I tell this story to my students. So, I filled my metal bucket with ice and placed it on my metal cart and started wheeling down the hall. I finally reached the end of the hall about 3 hours later, because I was socializing and talking with all of the patients. This was before DRGs and patients weren't as sick as they are now. They were happy to talk to someone new.

When I finally walked into the last room I looked at the patient and thought, 'She doesn't look so good to me.' I asked her if she'd like some ice in her water but she just lay there and didn't answer. I filled her pitcher anyway because she was on my list, but I made a little note on my paper to tell the nurse.

When I got back to the nurses' station I told her about the patient, but she brushed it off saying, "Oh, she's been dead a couple of hours." Now why would that nurse send me into that patient's room? I wasn't going to let her comment affect me so I replied, "Well, she was on my list so I put ice in her pitcher."

When I tell my students this story I laughingly tell them I knew I'd be a good nurse because I knew there was something wrong with that person. Did I know she was dead? No. Did I think to call someone right away? Not really, but I had good assessment skills because I knew that this patient didn't look like the rest of the people I was talking to. That's how I knew I was supposed to be a nurse!

What an eventful first day! Did you stay on that unit as a candy striper?

I did. I liked it there. The nurses were nice to me and I made friends. I stayed on that unit through high school, even though I could have moved to pediatrics or the nursery after a while.

I enrolled in a baccalaureate nursing program right out of high school, but just before I started taking nursing classes in my junior year I fell and broke my leg, fracturing the fibula and extending the tibia through the side of my leg. I needed 3 surgeries, and was on crutches and a cane for years. I took to wearing high top gym shoes because they gave me the best support for my ankle. It afforded me many funny stories because when I was in administrative positions I would wear power suits along with my bright pink high tops. That was before people wore their walking shoes to and from work, so I had a very unusual look.

What a terrible thing to happen, right at the start of your nursing career.

It was, but the worst part came when my dean called me and said that I should reconsider being a nurse because of my injury. "Nurses need legs that work," she told me, "and this is going to be very hard for you." At the time I thought she was extremely unsupportive, but I've come to think of it as one of those paradoxical interventions. Of course, she could have been telling me to quit, but I choose to believe that she was telling me to quit so that I'd get mad enough to show her that I wasn't going to.

I didn't quit, but I had to wear a brace for a long time. Later I switched to high tops, but always in a fun color. Never in black or anything low key.

When did you know in what area of nursing you'd like to practice?

I was always interested in psychiatric nursing and even minored in psychology in college. I know the reputation that psych nurses and psych instructors have, and with my background in both I wonder what that says about me! (laughter)

I didn't have a specific role model in school, but I did have a tough med/surg instructor who I liked. This was the beginning of nursing diagnoses, and among the handful of diagnoses available, only one dealt with psychosocial issues: Distress of the Human Spirit. I remember working with an oncology patient who was dying, but she was also being treated for several medical complications. My care plan listed Distress of the Human Spirit as her primary problem, and of course my instructor said, "I don't think so."

I argued with her that if the patient is dying and feels that we're unable to help her, then her number one problem is psychological. She immediately asked me if I wanted to be a psych nurse. I admitted that I had been thinking about it. "What a waste," she said. "You're smart and good with your medications. Why not choose another specialty?" She was encouraging me to go into oncology by telling me that these patients needed a great deal of psychosocial support as well, but I'd at least be working with medically ill patients. I never faulted her for her comments because I respected her as an instructor, even though she wasn't very much of a psych nurse.

It's funny how things come full-circle. Now, when my students try to choose the same diagnosis for medically complex patients in oncology, I tell them to pick something else. We talk about the psychosocial and spiritual issues affecting the patient, but there is another reason why the patient is in the hospital.

Did you work on a psychiatric unit after graduation?

I did. My first job was on a psych unit, which everyone tells you not to do. They recommend that you work in med/surg for a year and then specialize, but I was working in a well-respected medical center and the unit had many medically ill patients on the psych floor. There were patients with IVs and oxygen, and they did ECT (electroconvulsive therapy) right on the unit. Many patients were on tube feedings for eating disorders. We also had pregnant women on the unit because this was back when we had to discontinue psychotropic medications during pregnancy. So, we had many very sick schizophrenic or bipolar women who were in their third trimester. We went with them to the delivery room and helped them from a psychiatric point of view.

I gained a great deal of medical experience there even though it was a psych floor. I also learned the most about psychiatric nursing there because it was a teaching unit with residents, and supervision, and treatment planning.

Eventually I went back to school to become a psychiatric Clinical Nurse Specialist (CNS). I was drawn to child psych, where I believe there's more resilience and more possibility for change.

The perfect job for me showed up as a blind ad in the paper. They were looking for a master's level nurse doing therapy with adolescents, medication management, and crisis intervention. It sounded like a role I would have written myself. The ad didn't give the name of the facility though, and it took nearly the entire phone interview to find out that my employer would be a private corporation that had a contract with a maximum security prison. She offered me a generous salary, and told me I would be working with 12- to 18-year-old boys who had committed a felony, such as rape or murder, and have psychiatric illness.

This was my first job out of graduate school. I felt that if I could work with these kids, I could work with anyone. It was challenging though, especially for my family. My father was a Chicago cop and hated the idea. He couldn't believe that there weren't any other jobs out there for me.

He knew what working in a maximum security prison meant: signing a contract acknowledging that if you're ever taken hostage, they will not negotiate on your behalf, walking through 3 sets of locked gates to work each day, and not even being able to bring your own lunch to work. In this case, it's true what you see on TV. You eat in the cafeteria where the metal tray is your dish and the food is unceremoniously tossed onto your tray. That would be my lunch every day.

But I worked there for 3 years and enjoyed it.

What did you enjoy about it?

I liked working with the kids. Sure, they had done horrible things, but they had also had horrible lives. That was when I knew I would always have a job, because if this is how parents are bringing up children, or treating children, or ignoring children, there will always be a need for someone to work with kids and their families. We go through more education, training, and testing to drive a car than we do to raise a child. In fact, we don't mandate any education for child rearing. I don't know how enforceable it would be to do that, but there are a lot of people out there who are simply not prepared or capable to raise a child. And so there are unimaginably terrible things happening to a lot of these kids.

Is there someone you worked with who really stands out for you?

There are a couple, actually. One of the worst family stories I ever heard was about a young boy who was born to a very young (15- or 16-year-old) single girl whose mother didn't want her to have the baby. She wanted to keep the baby, but didn't have any prenatal care and drifted on the streets, and from friend to friend throughout her pregnancy until she had the baby prematurely. He was born with severe hearing loss and mild cerebral palsy.

She continued living on the streets after he was born, but in order to survive and keep the baby she joined the circus. It sounds unbelievable, but it's true. The first 3 or 4 years of this boy's life were spent traveling in a circus with a single mom who was barely 18 years of age.

Finally, the grandmother took some responsibility. She found her grandson and obtained proof that the mother wasn't capable of parenting, and she was able to keep him. It turned out that the grandmother wasn't the best caregiver either, and he wound up in 5 or 6 foster homes over the course of about 2 years. Around the time he was 7 years old his mother's sister took him in. She was married with 6 children of her own, and had a very solid family. He connected with his cousins and the parents were very loving toward him.

One day this boy and his aunt and a few of the children were crossing the street, and the aunt was struck by a car and was killed instantly. His aunt was the only person who ever treated him kindly and she was killed before his eyes. The husband couldn't manage all of the children alone and sent this boy back to foster care.

This child's life was a series of tragedies and disruptions. It's no wonder that he quickly wound up in jail and was sent to a youth detention center. It was here that he was accused of raping another boy. He said he didn't do it, and I really believed him. I know that everyone says they didn't do it, but there was something about the way he said it that made me believe him.

His story becomes more tragic. He ran away from the center because he believed even though he didn't commit the crime, he was still going to be punished for it. The more he thought about getting in trouble for something he didn't do, the more he convinced himself that he might as well commit the crime. He found a little boy on the street and raped him. Now he has 2 rape charges against him and he is sent to prison.

The crime he admits to is the second rape. How can you expect that this young man would ever turn into anything but a problem?

I was able to form a therapeutic relationship with him and I could see that he was caring toward me. He would worry about me when there were other boys around who were more aggressive or more threatening, and he would advise me not to talk to certain people because they weren't safe. I could see how he could form an attachment, but he just never had that opportunity, in his whole life, to forge that connection with someone. He never learned right from wrong, or how to be nice to people without being assaultive or aggressive. His was such a sad story and he really touched my life.

There was another boy I worked with who was very, very sick. I think he was probably hearing voices and had a lot of mental health issues from a very young age. He was always trying to kill himself and doing crazy things to end his life because he was in so much pain. I really connected with him, too.

I worked with him until he turned 18. He was so sick, clearly, that he wound up in other mental health hospitals instead of staying in prison. I always knew where he was being transferred because he would send me letters each time he was about to be placed in seclusion or in restraints in one of these facilities. The patient has the right to inform someone of a change in circumstances and he would always use my name. That's really against the rules, though. You are not supposed to have any communication with the prisoners when they are outside of your facility. Every now and again I'd be called into the superintendent's office and I would tell them to just open the letter and see for themselves that I wasn't communicating with anyone. They'd then see that it was a form letter from the mental health facility stating that this young man had been restrained again.

It touched my heart that this young man had absolutely no one in his life, and that in his confused thinking I was the only one he thought would want to know that he was being placed in restraints. He didn't have a single friend or family member to tell.

Obviously, you were the only one he felt any closeness to in this world. Do you think you were able to help him while he was seeing you?

I do think that I helped him learn how to live with his illness. Medication can help, but it won't fix the problem. Much of the work that psychiatric nurses do with people who have chronic mental illness is in problem solving and coping strategies. I think when people have the experience of receiving unconditional positive regard from someone, especially when they've never had it, it allows them to have a relationship in a positive way. We always hope that our work translates for them in their life with other people.

It's about lending out your ego. As a healthy person doing therapy, you're giving yourself to them and allowing them to see how you're experiencing something. Then they can start asking, "What would Maryan do right now?" Hopefully over time, they would integrate that and it would become part of how they change their behavior. I hope I was able to accomplish that for my patients.

Earlier you referred to a certain reputation that psychiatric nurses have. Can you elaborate on that?

I don't think that a reputation is warranted for any specialty area. There is good and bad in every area. The problem is the majority of people who are good and caring and do a good job aren't really that interesting. It doesn't make for good TV drama or movie characters. I do think there are people out there who are like Nurse Ratched and I think there are crazy cat ladies as psychiatric nurses, but that's not the majority and it's never warranted to use stereotypes.

What made you leave the prison?

When you work in psychiatry and give so much of yourself in your interactions, you're at a big risk of burning out, which is what happened to me. I tell my students that you are your therapeutic tool, and you should be taking excellent care of yourself. You wouldn't tie your stethoscope in a knot and throw it in your trunk at the end of your shift. My family saw how the job was affecting me and with their encouragement I eventually left the prison and entered into the private sector in program development and administrative roles.

Let's fast-forward to your current position as a nursing instructor in an associate degree program. Tell me about this role.

There was a long time in my life that I never thought I would teach. I didn't have the right role models in nursing school. Remember the old adage, "Those who can't—teach"? Well, we certainly believed that about many of our nursing instructors, and teaching didn't appeal to me early on in my career.

I've always been a workaholic in every job I had and when I hit a significant decade marker about 8 years ago, I started to reevaluate priorities in my life and my career. I thought teaching would allow me a better balance in my life. This was a huge change for me. I've worked at very prestigious public and private hospitals across the country, and have degrees from prominent private universities, and I place a very high value on higher education. However, I needed to make a change in my career and I decided to answer a small ad in the *Nursing Spectrum* for a part-time psychiatric nurse instructor, which I later learned was located at a community college in my neighborhood.

I accepted the position of adjunct clinical instructor. It was a 6-week course that met on Saturdays and Sundays, which worked for me because I worked Monday through Friday at the hospital. My workload certainly didn't lessen, but I eventually left my full-time position for extended hours at the college. That led to an offer to teach a med/surg course. I had never even been a med/surg nurse, but I did have medical experience in acute psych. I reviewed the materials and studied a great deal and thoroughly enjoyed it. They made me an offer to join the program and I accepted.

I was very happy with my decision, but my friends couldn't believe that I would teach in a community college. I am very proud, though, of my nursing program. The instructors are extremely dedicated and we have an excellent reputation among schools of nursing. What didn't quite work out is that I am still working 60 hours a week. I don't even have the summers off because I'm either teaching or taking classes myself. My heart is in nursing, but I still struggle with finding a balance.

The big issue today is the pending shortage of nurses, and it's finally reaching the public that the shortage has as much, if not more, to do with a lack of faculty than with the number of nursing school applicants. What are your thoughts?

I agree, and I think the bigger issue is the funding of faculty. I left a healthy 6-figure income for an annual salary of $40,000 as a first year full-time faculty member. A master's level nurse teaching at the college is paid the same as someone with a master's in English, who's straight out of graduate school, teaching communication. It isn't that they're not valuable, because we need people to teach our students, but should they be paid the same as someone who's worked for 20 years as a nurse and who has completely different responsibilities with students? I take my students to the hospital and we provide all of the care for our patients. There is a difference between overseeing clinical practice and helping a student in the classroom.

Another perspective on faculty salaries is to look at the $26 per hour that a college pays an adjunct faculty, which is less than or equal to what our nursing students are paid upon graduation. I think teachers and nurses are undervalued overall in society, so a nursing teacher takes a double hit. How can you keep good people when you are not paying them appropriately?

After salary, the next issue is clinical site availability. We're saturated with schools in this area and we're all competing for the same clinical sites. We're being creative by working weekends and evenings, but we still don't have enough locations. We might be able to hire more faculty, and we could certainly admit more students, but we don't have the clinical sites to accommodate them.

We need better, more collaborative partnerships between hospitals and nursing schools by implementing teacher-practitioner roles (working 2 days in the hospital and 3 days at the school). The hospital would contribute to the teacher's salary and the school would have a consistent clinical location.

I'd like to bring up the age-old issue of ADN versus BSN and entry into practice. How do you weigh in?

I have my BSN and I do think that the BSN is extremely valuable, but I'm very proud of the education I provide to my nursing students at the community college level. If I had it to do over again today I would absolutely get my ADN first and start working. Hospitals are offering very generous tuition reimbursement programs and other creative ways to obtain a BSN and I would take advantage of that.

A baccalaureate degree is very important in nursing, but I don't think it has to be entry level. I would challenge anyone to come to one of my units and observe ADN nurses and BSN nurses working side by side, and tell me by watching them who is the BSN and who is the ADN nurse.

Can we look at this from another perspective? Do you think we have the right type of educational programs to prepare nurses for entry into practice? Rather than look at an associate degree versus a baccalaureate degree, do you think there might be a hybrid program that would meet our needs?

That's a very good question. I do think that programs are changing, which the NLN has called for. I'm on the curriculum committee and we are in the process of updating our nursing program. We have been very content heavy and much of our teaching has been connected to the medical model. We'll be using Marjorie Gordon for our organizational framework and we're going to work from a nursing perspective and concentrate on critical thinking, prioritization, and the things that fall into the nursing realm.

Maybe we need to take a look at the role hospitals play in the transition from school to work as well. Here's a real opportunity for some partnering with hospitals and other locations where new grads will be working. I think schools are trying to look at real world practice, but it's when you're actually in practice that you're finally experiencing those issues.

We should also look at formal preceptor and mentor programs, and reimburse the nurse preceptors. What I see are the same few good nurses who always volunteer to be preceptors, but they eventually burn out. The reality is there's a staffing crunch, so the nurses' case load will not be lowered, and there will be days when someone calls in sick and you'll have to cover. How can that be done when you are supposed to be nurturing and developing a new nurse? What are we saying about how we value our nurses, if we don't allow for a more formalized transition into practice?

Is there a particular story or experience that you've had as a teacher that makes you proud of this career choice?

I clearly feel that this is the right place for me to be, and I'm happiest when I'm with the students. I feel like I'm making a difference. I'm creating good nurses. I have very high expectations and I have a reputation at school for being tough, but I also have students come back and tell me that they learned so much from me and that they're glad they had me as an instructor.

There are moments every day that make me proud of my students, but I had a really wonderful experience last semester. Things happened that made me think, "It was meant to be."

I'm a huge advocate of education and continuing education programs. I'm currently enrolled in graduate education classes, and I try to attend seminars that apply clinically to my work. Last semester I attended a program sponsored by the hospital where I have clinical privileges. They have a fabulous cardiology program and the seminar identified the latest protocol in cardiac assessment for patients presenting to the emergency department with specific cardiac signs and symptoms.

Two weeks after attending the seminar I had a group of nursing students at that hospital and one was taking care of a patient who was starting to have the very same non-descript changes that they talked about in my seminar. The stars were aligned because the student nurse had only one patient, which we all know never happens (1:1 nurse-patient ratio) outside of a critical care unit, and noticed these changes. She was also a very good student and alert enough to notify me and the staff nurse so that the staff nurse could complete her own assessment and order a stat EKG. Sure enough, the EKG had some of the changes that I learned about in the seminar just 2 weeks before.

Why did I choose that patient for my student? Certainly not for any cardiac purpose. The patient didn't even have a cardiac history, but those ST changes clearly indicated a need for immediate intervention. The cardiologist looked at the results and told us to get this patient into the cath lab right away, but not before he thanked us for following through on this great assessment.

I think we saved this woman's life. It was a string of lucky coincidences and everything fell into place. I happened to attend a seminar on my day off from work, which was not being reimbursed by my employer, but because that's my value system I went and I paid attention. Two weeks later I chose 1 patient out of 40 for this student to follow. It was as if a guardian angel helped me pick this patient. Her student nurse was sharp enough to notice the changes, and my relationship with the staff nurses was good enough that they respected my clinical judgment and contacted the cardiologist.

Everything went smoothly with this patient, but here's the part I love best. My student accompanied the patient to the cath lab and after a short conversation with the nurse there realized that the cath lab nurse was my former student from my first semester of teaching! That was 8 years ago. They exchanged stories while the patient was being prepped for the procedure, and my current student noticed the medications that were being drawn. She told the group, "This patient is allergic to codeine," but no one paid attention. She interrupted again, and this time my former student added, "You know, this is Jatczak's student and she probably knows the right information. I would have needed to know the same information as her student, so let's take a stop and double check."

They double checked, and found that my student was correct and probably prevented another problem from occurring. The doctor actually called to thank me for choosing this patient in the first place and to let me know how much he appreciated having me as part of their team.

I'm only at that hospital one shift per week, and so many good things fell into place for this patient in that short period of time. I'm so proud of what we all did, and until the actual moment when the doctor began the procedure it was all nursing.

We made a difference in this patient's life and the thing is.... she has no clue. She was already failing fast in the elevator, and won't remember our faces, much less our names, but that's not what's important. That's how nurses touch patients. It's not about memorizing medications but having the critical thinking capability to understand the larger picture. It's about relationship building, knowledge, values, confidence, and more. For me, it's a story that holds so much meaning on so many levels. It also makes me think that I was meant to be at that seminar.

Your story almost makes this next question anticlimactic, but do you consider your work to be heroic?

No. I've never considered myself heroic, ever. Making a decision to call a doctor about a patient assessment doesn't take courage...it's what nurses do.

Maryan Jatczak, MSN, BSN
Assistant Professor of Nursing
Illinois

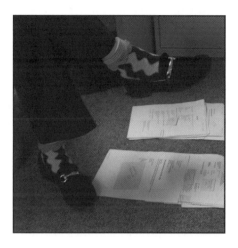

CHAPTER 37

And the Oscar Goes to...

Did you know early on that you would choose nursing as a career?

No, never. Nursing wasn't my first career choice, and I was already a mature woman when I entered the profession. I realized in the early 1980s that I was going to have to go back to work. It was around the time when I was visiting my sister in the hospital, who was very, very sick. I spent a lot of time with her and would see nurses sitting around the nurses' station and whizzing in and out of patient rooms. I thought, "This is something I could do." It was never a Mother Theresa moment. Not at all.

This was pre-DRGs (diagnosis-related groups) when a patient's length of stay in the hospital wasn't strictly regulated.

That's right. So I went to nursing school and graduated with an associate degree in the late 1980s. I immediately applied to a major medical center because they offered college tuition reimbursement for employees and their children. I thought it was a great deal because I had college-aged children who could benefit from the program.

I was disappointed initially, because they were looking for nurses with BSNs, but I was pushy and kept asking for an interview. Finally, one of the nurse managers agreed to interview me. When she called to offer me the job she said, "I always go with the underdogs." And I thought, "Now I'm an underdog? I always thought I was an upper-dog!"

I stayed there 4 years, but it was difficult work. I was on a surgical unit, and we saw a variety of very complicated cases, from radical neck surgeries to hip and knee replacements, to urological surgeries and more. These were patients who spent 24 hours in intensive care and were transferred to our unit. Patients were sick and they were in pain. Today we have PCA (patient controlled analgesia) pumps where patients are able to self-administer regulated doses of pain medication intravenously, but back then we ran up and down the halls giving Demerol injections, which wasn't nearly as effective.

Did you ever find out why your manager considered you an underdog?

Because I didn't have a BSN. In the 1980s hospitals were hiring a lot of bachelor's degree nurses and I had an associate degree. As I said, I was a mature woman and didn't look like a typical new grad nurse; the residents would equate age with number of years in practice and would always come to me with their questions. Lo and behold, I always seemed to have the answers they wanted, so I fit right in, but it was always a struggle. I worked the evening shift and it was actually a good night when I got home at 1:30 in the morning. Those days have never left me.

When I recruit new grads I always feel a bit of compassion for them, knowing what they'll be facing. Nursing is a difficult profession, and it is a huge responsibility to know you are that patient's advocate for the next 8 or 12 hours.

There were good days too. The camaraderie with my coworkers made it feel very much like a family. And there were the patients whom you never forgot as well.

Is there anyone who stands out for you?

Yes, one does, and she had flaming red hair. She was a very beautiful woman. I remember she came in on a Sunday afternoon. Her nails were polished and her hair was done and she looked stunning. Very often patients would come in on the PM shift the day before their surgery. She had throat cancer and was going to have radical neck surgery. I knew she wouldn't be able to speak for a very long time, if ever, after that surgery, and from the way she spoke to the resident after signing her consent form, I just knew she didn't know what was in store for her.

I believe the patient should always know what is going to happen next. It is a promise I developed, and I didn't learn it in school. It was obvious this patient didn't know what to expect. I didn't want to scare her by any means, but I wanted to talk with her and let her know what she could anticipate after surgery. I called the resident back, who explained everything for her in greater detail. She wasn't as happy afterward but she was knowledgeable. I don't know what her long-term prognosis was, but she did very well after surgery and ultimately was discharged home.

I eventually left that hospital and went into management. I was the clinical director for a nonprofit health care organization, and we had the best mission statement that I could ever have hoped for. Our mission was to take care of people who did not have health care insurance. These people were working 2 and 3 jobs just to make ends meet, but they didn't have insurance; yet we took care of them—no questions asked. It was so fulfilling to work there, but after a few years my position lost its funding, so I had to find a new job.

What prompted you to go into management?

I pursued a bachelor's degree in nursing and then continued on to graduate school. I took the management route because I was older, and because the only other alternative was to become a Clinical Nurse Specialist (CNS). There was a certain amount of confusion surrounding advanced nursing degrees back then, and people were saying there weren't any jobs out there for CNSs. Nurse Practitioners (NPs) were just gaining recognition, but we weren't clear about how the NP's role differed from the CNS's role. The clearest career path for nurses with graduate degrees was for those pursuing a master's degree in nursing administration.

I fear history is repeating itself with the advent of the Clinical Nurse Leader (CNL) designation. This is another graduate nursing degree, but I don't know how the Nurse Leader's role differs from the Nurse Manager's role. I know that there is a place for them, but in the meantime I see some role confusion by introducing another level of nurse. I am now a Nurse Recruiter and I haven't seen many ads for a Clinical Nurse Leader.

From your vantage point as a Nurse Recruiter, are you affected at all by the nursing shortage?

No, I don't notice it at all. I work for the federal government and we see a steady stream of resumés. What I do notice is that people do not want to be managers. Management positions are very difficult to fill. Long-term care is another very difficult area.

Hospital administrators need to acknowledge that nursing is a darn hard job. There are intrinsic rewards in nursing, but there should also be financial compensation. Nurses are not nuns and they should be compensated fairly for their work. I'd also like to see the hospital sponsor certifications and continuing education credits for those nurses practicing in geriatrics. It would be a great way to redefine the image of long-term care. They could also provide more leadership development programs for managers.

Any physician will say that nurses have a tough road. I've worked with many surgeons and believe me, they want the best nurses taking care of their patients. They don't want to see their work in the OR go awry. Think about it. Why is the patient in the hospital? They're in the hospital because they're receiving 24-hour care from a nurse. If we didn't have nurses on duty why would there be hospitals?

You've experienced several roles as a registered nurse, from staff nurse to management and now to recruitment. Would you consider any of your work, in any role, to be heroic?

No.

That was fast.

Emphatically no.

Why is that?

I think of heroes as life savers, and I don't think I've ever saved anybody's life. I think I helped them, and might have made their evening or night a little bit easier. I always try to do the right thing but no, I wouldn't say I was heroic. A heroic nurse is someone who answers codes or is flying in helicopters overseas with our servicemen and women. There are plenty of heroic nurses around, but I don't think I'm one of them. I don't even think I belong in this book, to tell you the truth.

I always enjoy hearing nurses' comments to this question, and it's always a resounding answer, whether it's yes or no. I would say that the response I get is 50/50, and even when the answer is yes, many times the nurse wonders why his or her story warrants a place in this book. I think those responses validate the title.

I know that not everyone can be a nurse, though. Nurses take care of people when they can't do things—intimate things—for themselves. I think that is one way that nurses stand out. I can remember taking care of my father when he was sick, and trying to help him in the bathroom. My presence made him so uncomfortable, and he'd wince, "Oh Joan, can you please just get out of here! I don't want you doing this for me." And I'd reply, "Pa, I do this for strangers, why wouldn't I do it for you?" He just didn't like that idea at all! "You mean you do this for strange men?" he'd grumble. I can laugh about it now, but he thought that was terrible. This is what nurses do, though.

I can remember taking care of another older gentleman who was admitted through the ER. He wasn't homeless, but he was just filthy, poor guy. He didn't have anyone to take care of him at home. We were simply aghast when we saw him. We couldn't even put him in bed, so I told him he'd have to take a shower. I brought him to the shower room and had him sit down, while I got a clean plastic bag from the garbage can and used it to cover myself. I can remember washing his feet and he looked down at me and said in all sincerity, "You know honey, you've really got a lousy job." I looked at him and laughed, "You know, I never thought of it that way, but you've got a point there!"

But again, you're doing intimate things for people. I don't think everyone can do this.

They don't prepare you for every circumstance in nursing school, but I do think that there has to be a portion of you that can be an actress. You have to remain calm and collected even when your instructor is questioning you in front of your patient. You also have to keep your composure when you're in emergency situations or negotiating with physicians. I was much older when I went to nursing school, so I think that having had children and just the wisdom of my years helped me through those situations. I marvel at the young people in school today and think, 'I couldn't have done that when I was their age.' My hat's off to them. Now, those young people are already heroes, in my opinion.

Joan Flynn, MSN, RN
Nurse Recruiter
Illinois

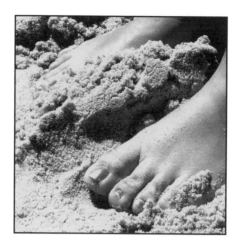

CHAPTER 38

A Little Luxury Called Time

I knew exactly where I wanted to work and they hired me...eventually.

When I first applied to the National Institutes of Health (NIH), they declined my application. I had a bachelor's degree in biology and an associate degree in nursing and I wanted to combine my background in biology with nursing, and do research. I attended an open house and the nurse recruiter asked, "What is your PhD in?" I shook my head, "No." "Okay," she continued, "what is your master's degree in?" Again I replied in the negative. "Well," she asked, "do you have a bachelor's degree?" Finally I could say, "Yes. I have a BS in biology and an AD in nursing." But they weren't hiring non-baccalaureate prepared nurses at that time. So, I went to work in another hospital as a staff nurse in oncology.

You started as a biology major. How did you become involved in nursing?

After graduating I worked in an environmental lab doing waste water analysis, because you couldn't do anything with a biology degree if you weren't teaching or going to medical school. I had two colleagues at the lab, one was studying for his MCATs to become an MD and the other was studying for her NCLEX to become an RN. I remember looking through their books and being much more interested in the nursing questions.

My local community college had a nursing program that had a very good reputation, so I enrolled and graduated in 2 years. I had the option of attending an accelerated 18-month baccalaureate program, but I also had a mortgage to pay and that program was too intense to complete while working full time.

There are decades-long debates about a standardized entry into nursing practice. Would you like to weigh in?

I have very strong opinions about that, absolutely. I've always felt that education provides a blueprint of how to start an IV, interpret an EKG, or assess a patient, but the actual building materials are what we individually bring to practice—that being our own personal experiences, our backgrounds, even our personalities. Clearly I value education, as I've worked my way up the educational ladder, having just finished my master's program. But I also started my nursing career as an AD nurse—and never once did I feel inferior in any way to my colleagues holding a BSN. I never felt under-prepared, or at a disadvantage. I think that the term "entry level nurse" is just that—it's the entry point into the profession. As with any profession, there's room for growth—both personal and educational. AD nurses have all the necessary skills required to be a Registered Nurse. Where you take your education beyond that "entry level" is up to the individual.

Maybe this is the wrong argument to have, and instead of debating which nurse is better prepared, we should

be looking at a completely different model for entry into practice. I don't know what that would look like, but it might be a hybrid of existing programs, with easy access to graduate programs.

I completely agree. Something has to give, and I'm guessing it will be influenced by the baby boom generation. The emphasis should be on whether or not a patient is getting good, competent nursing care, not on how many degrees and letters nurses have behind their names.

How did you get involved in oncology and then gerontology?

The biggest fears I had growing up were hospitals and cancer. I was absolutely terrified. And I wound up in a hospital, working with oncology patients. I think that the more afraid you are of something the more you read and learn about it. Because I was always an information seeker, I learned as much as I could about cancer. The real clincher though, was walking into the room of a woman who was dying. She was sitting there just looking out the window, and being so thankful that she was able to watch the sun come up. She said, "You just don't understand how grateful you are for every morning until you're faced with the fact you might not see another morning tomorrow." I will never forget that moment. As a student, it had a huge impact on the way I started to view things.

I was also tremendously influenced by my grandparents as I was growing up. I have such a love and reverence for the elderly because my dad's parents were around so much of the year and I spent a lot of time with them. They would come and visit, and tell stories. I found it very rewarding.

So I combined my love for the elderly with oncology and completed a dual Nurse Practitioner (NP) program in geriatric oncology. Two-thirds of individuals with cancer are over the age of 55, which is defined as geriatrics. But here I am, doing something different again.

Did you work as a nurse practitioner?

No, not really. For my current position as a Research Coordinator they wanted a master's prepared nurse, but I'm not prescribing right now.

Do you miss not working as a nurse practitioner?

You know what I don't miss quite honestly? I don't miss being on call. I talk to my colleagues who are working as NPs and they describe their days of high anxiety and low self-esteem. And these are brilliant women. They're working 12- and 14-hour days, but they're not able to provide the kind of care they're used to providing as very conscientious practitioners, and they're scared about losing their licenses. Many of them are in long-term care facilities and have shared with me that they feel their collaborating physicians are not providing them with the necessary back up, feedback, constructive criticism, and mentorship that they need as new practitioners, and they're having very difficult transitions.

They just look at me and shake their heads saying, "You've got the golden goose." And I would have to agree with them.

A lot of my friends who completed the geriatric NP program are working for companies that offer special needs plans for people who are Medicare/Medicaid eligible. The patient enrolls in this type of plan and receives a range of health care services. These patients are usually in long-term care facilities and the companies follow a "treat in place" model as opposed to treating the patients in a hospital.

From what my friends have told me, the vast majority of patients are DNRs. I don't want to say they're coerced, but having a DNR is strongly recommended. The NPs have caseloads between 70 and 80 patients per nursing home, and some of them have 2 to 3 nursing homes. They see each patient monthly, and deal with acute issues as they arise. But my overall impression is that frequently, NPs are on an assembly line and they're simply seeing a set number of patients during a set period of time.

I said to my dad that there's nothing more sad and depressing than a nursing home. By this I mean that so many special people are "warehoused" and put away to live out the remainder of their lives in solitude, under-stimulated and under-valued. I started to get involved with a nonprofit organization he's been involved with called Partners in Care, which helps older and disabled adults remain independent in their own homes. People volunteer their time and give back to the community. It's a great concept because they believe everyone has something to contribute and is valued for it. I sat in on a few of their board meetings but I don't have the time to commit to it right now. But this long-term care landscape is very concerning to me.

On another note, I shadowed the Dean of my school who works part time as the nurse practitioner for a continuing care retirement community. Talk about a different world! It was built for people who are in a higher income bracket, and it was simply spectacular. But most people can't afford that. Most people are going to get warehoused. And it's only going to be once the baby boomers start getting into these situations that things will change. It's going to take a mass movement to improve health care for the elderly.

How did you make your way back to NIH?

The first time I applied at NIH I thought it would be a neat coupling of nursing and biology. You're not exposed to research in school, but I thought it would be experimental and cutting edge, and exciting. The second time around I had my experience in oncology nursing to offer, and I knew they did a lot of cancer research. My aunt had died at a young age from a brain tumor and I was interested in the newest treatments and experimental procedures that other hospitals weren't doing.

I had worked for 18 months on an inpatient adult surgical oncology unit. I developed my clinical skills there. There were always tubes, and drains, and wounds, and chemo. And there were a lot of spiritual aspects to the work that I became very comfortable with. I'm very interested in aging and spirituality. As nurses, we spend a lot of time trying to master the clinical skills so we can concentrate on the people aspect of healing someone—not just physically, but emotionally and spiritually.

Can you think of an instance where this came together for you?

I can think of a really good experience and a really bad one, and they both occurred about the same time. Let's start with the bad one. I was a new nurse working with a gentleman whose family was hovering, waiting for him to die. He had coded multiple times after dialysis and it became a common occurrence. This had gone on for some time, and I remember that he had drifted into a semi-conscious state. His family meanwhile, was outside of his room, angry and bickering and fighting about money. I can remember it got to the point where they knew he was dying and probably wasn't going to pull out of it this time—and everybody left! They just left him there. I remember going into his room and taking vitals, and trying to comfort him, but none of his family remained.

I had walked into his room with another nurse and I can remember watching him. He was just barely there—and then he wasn't. But at the last minute he sat straight up in bed and screamed at the top of his lungs. He was in a place that was not good, and then he lay down and that was it. He was gone. I can remember the hair on the back of my neck stood up. That was a bad death. That was one of my introductions to the idea that there are good deaths and bad deaths, and then there are just deaths. That is one of the only real negative dying experiences that I've had.

On a totally different note, I can remember an older woman who was dying of breast cancer. She had been slipping, and slipping. Two of her daughters were at her bedside, but she was hanging on, trying to wait for a third daughter to fly in from the west coast.

I can remember the woman just barely hanging on, until her third daughter finally arrived and was able to say goodbye. The patient was unconscious, but she had tears coming out of her eyes. I can remember the 3 daughters sitting around their mom's bed singing that old camp song, "Make new friends, but keep the old, One is silver, the other is gold." They were singing in a round melody as their mom passed.

We could hear those angelic voices coming from her room and it was just very emotional for everybody on the ward. It was a good passing. Her daughter was able to make it there in time and the patient had held on. You see it over and over. You definitely choose your time.

I've also experienced 2 very good passings with my grandparents. I'm not a religious person, but I am a very spiritual person and I think having those positive experiences and being around good people and watching them go through the motions of dealing with a terminal diagnosis really impact you. If you think you're having a bad day, let me introduce you to one of my patients. I don't always live by that, but I try. Sometimes, they pop into my mind at really weird times. It probably happens with most nurses. You might be walking along a beautiful place or quiet area and all of a sudden somebody pops into your head, and you think, "That was 7 years ago! Where did that come from?"

I think that I have really learned a lot about who I am through my experiences and talking with patients. One of the greatest things I loved about NIH was our patient-to-nurse ratio. A normal patient load on an adult med/surg oncology unit would be 3 patients on the day shift, 3 patients on evenings and 3 to 4 on nights.

Tell me about your new job.

I now work for the National Institute of Environmental Health Sciences (NIEHS). It's a small group based out of the Research Triangle in North Carolina, but we're physically located on the NIH campus. I'm the Research Coordinator for the Environmental Autoimmunity Group. Currently, the protocol we are working on recruits pediatric and adult myositis patients. Myositis is an inflammatory autoimmune condition of the muscle. It's not like cancer where you know the end outcome, in many cases. Myositis has more of a smoldering effect, with flare-ups and remissions, and debilitating weakness, but no known cure.

I'm coordinating a Phase I double-blinded placebo controlled randomized trial, which is the highest integrity of protocol there is. It's a much more administrative focus than what I have been doing but it's really interesting to see the flip side of the research. I'm listed as an associate investigator, which means I'll be involved in documenting results and writing reports for the public.

Some people reading this will think that's a cake walk.

Some days it is and some days it's hell, depending on what kind of research protocol they are on, and if you are doing serial blood draws every 5 minutes, and you are responsible for implementing Phase 1 intraperitoneal chemotherapy dwells—where they are instilling warmed hemo into bellies, sewing them up, and sending them back to the floor. Everything that happens must be documented. You never have any idea if, for instance, the patient is hallucinating because he has cancer or because you just gave him an experimental dose of a new medication.

Most days you could sit down in a chair and talk to a patient one-on-one about life, how they came to your floor, how they feel about where they are going, or about end of life. You get close to these people. And there are so many amazing stories and life events you take away and you just kind of house them all and draw on them throughout your nursing career and throughout your own life.

We also had support on the unit. The palliative care team would have a brown bag lunch session with the nurses every 3 to 4 weeks. It was like a grieving session because the nurses needed an outlet. The patients who came to our ward usually had 6 months or less to live. It was just incredible. My drive time to work was about 45 minutes; driving in, I would listen to the radio and decompress, but driving home, there were many nights I cried for 45 minutes straight, but then I'd walk in the house and was fine. I have mentored new nurses who were so embarrassed when I found them sobbing after having lost their first patient, but they have to grieve. I've told them that if they don't grieve, they can't give back. They have to continue and they've got a life to live as well.

Because of the title of this book, I've been asking nurses if they consider their work to be heroic. How would you respond to that question?

Wow. Heroic. That's such a strong word, but if I've been able to give something of myself in that nature, it would be that I was present with someone while they were dying. I think that sitting at a patient's bedside, holding his or her hand, and comforting the family is an incredibly intimate moment in someone's life. You're not asked to show sympathy and the family doesn't want you to sit there and cry with them. They just want your strength and support.

I don't think nurses realize what an impact they have until we get notes back from patients, or somebody comes back to see you on the 1-year anniversary of their husband's death and brings in a peace lily.

Have you had that happen?

Oh yes. Many times family members will come back in tears and tell you that you've made such an impact on their lives. There was a woman whose sister had died and she came back to our unit with a little peace lily. She was in tears and could barely say thank you. She had a picture of her sister and had a thank you note from her entire family about what a difference it was to have people around who knew how to deal with her passing.

There's nothing worse, though, than having to say goodbye to a patient that you know is going home to die. I remember one gentleman very distinctly. He was my age and we became very close. We had done everything we could for him, but he knew he was going home to die. NIH is a place of last resort. I can remember him calling me into his room, sitting down on the bed with his arms around me—just sobbing. He was going home to die and he knew it. It was all he could do to thank me and everybody else for being there; for being supportive and understanding, listening to him gripe and complain, and just reminding him he's a person.

These experiences are all so bittersweet. You've made lasting impressions on so many people, which must feel rewarding, but they're heart-wrenching at the same time.

There's one more interesting story that I'll tell you and it goes back to taking the time to sit down and actually talk to a patient. I believe it really changed this man's treatment, and possibly his life. He was about 50 years old and was coming in for prostate surgery. He had horrendously high blood pressure. I can remember sitting down with him one day when I had some time on my hands and said, "Okay, let's look at your medications." So I took out all of his medications and placed them on his bed, and we reviewed everything.

He told me about the oral blood pressure medications he had transitioned through, and now he was using the highest dosage level of clonidine patch, but his blood pressure was still uncontrollable.

I was getting him ready for surgery and needed to know when he had last applied his patch. He was to apply it every three days and I wanted to make sure we had the same dosage available, so I asked him to show me one of his patches. Clonidine patches look like nicotine patches. They're small discs of medication, with an overlay of foam rubber adhesive. He pulled out his box of patches and handed me the foam rubber adhesive.

I remember that I sat there for a few minutes and finally said, "Mr. Smith, I need to talk with you about this medication. You've just handed me what goes over your clonidine patch." And he said, "No, Anna. That is the clonidine patch." And I tried to tell him that nowhere on that portion did it indicate the dosage level; it was just the adhesive. I asked him what he did with the other piece—the medication—and he told me he thought that was the cover and he had thrown them all away.

For 3½ years, this well-educated gentleman was opening each packet, throwing out the medicated disc and applying the foam rubber adhesive to his arm. He had gone through $15,000 worth of medication and had essentially thrown it all away.

He turned purple; he yelled. And it wasn't because he was an angry man. It was because for 3 years his health had deteriorated, probably as a result of his uncontrolled hypertension. And no one could figure it out.

He was livid. "Why couldn't my Ivy League educated cardiologist tell me how to apply this patch properly?" he yelled. His doctor might have looked at the patch, but there was always another adhesive over it, and you would assume that the disc was present. No one had ever looked underneath.

My concern was, of course, here we are 3 years later on the highest level of clonidine patch you can give a patient and if he goes to surgery and we apply another patch his blood pressure will bottom out. I notified his attending physician and called for a cardiology consult immediately. I didn't know if we would have to postpone his surgery until we could start treating him for his hypertension.

Having had the time to sit down and talk with this patient changed his whole course of treatment. Time isn't a luxury anymore. It's essential.

Anna V. Engstrom, RN, MS, GNP-BC
Research Nurse Specialist, Environmental Autoimmunity Group
Maryland

CHAPTER 39

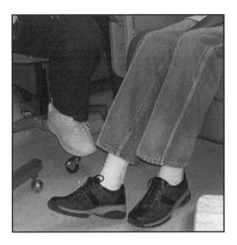

Fighting the Good Fight

W hen I graduated from nursing school in 1988, I applied for a nursing position at the hospital where I worked as a nursing assistant. They had 2 vacancies and asked me to choose between 2 units. I chose oncology. There wasn't any magic to my decision, but looking back, I know that I wouldn't have been happy in any other area. This is where I was meant to be.

What have you learned from your oncology patients over the years?

Many of our patients are older and have a very strong belief system. Their faith in God helps them to prepare both emotionally and spiritually, so we encourage them to talk about their beliefs in the clinic. I believe that they have much better outcomes because they don't have as much fear.

It seems like you have a very close-knit community here.

We do. Our team is wonderful and we always work in partnership with our doctors. You would never imagine it, but we actually have a lot of fun in our clinic! We turn on the television first thing in the morning and watch Oprah and talk about celebrities while the patients snack on food they've brought from home. We don't do any crying or feeling sorry for ourselves here, in fact we actually spend a lot of time laughing! You wouldn't think you could do that in an oncology setting, but we do.

We are very giving with our patients, and they are giving in return. On the morning of 9/11, we were all watching television in the clinic while I was starting an IV on my patient. Everyone was stunned by what we saw and many of us were crying. As I was starting my patient's IV on one hand, he was rubbing my shoulder to comfort me with the other. We all help each other here.

Are there any patients who stand out for you?

I remember one patient who was only 20 years old when she was diagnosed with acute leukemia. She was an undocumented alien who came here for treatment, and we took care of her. She was such a tiny, little thing and didn't speak much English, but she always had a smile on her face— even when she was sick. We fought alongside her for more than a year to save her life, but we didn't win the battle. Toward the end we knew there was nothing more that we could do for her. That's when she told us that she wanted to go back home to Mexico. So, the staff in the clinic and the hospital took up a collection to help offset her travel costs. She was home for nearly 2 weeks before she finally succumbed to her illness. She and her family were very grateful for everything the hospital and staff did for her. This was 3 years ago, and the family still sends postcards.

We've also taken up collections for patients who don't have health insurance. If we're giving chemotherapy but the patient can't afford the anti-nausea medication, the staff will pitch in so that the patient can buy his medication. That's just how we work here.

As a nurse, would you consider your actions to be heroic?

I wouldn't say that. You do what needs to be done. I do for my patients what I would want someone to do for me. We're here to care for them, and we'll do our very best to do just that.

Alritta Hubbard, RN
Staff Nurse, Outpatient Chemotherapy
Illinois

CHAPTER 40

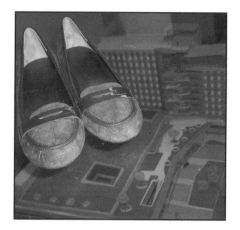

Hospital of the Future

T here are so many exciting things happening at Palomar Pomerado Health (PPH). I have been here 22 years and started as a staff nurse in critical care. I was the chief nurse for Palomar Medical Center in 2000, and in 2004 I became the chief nurse for the entire health care system. It's been quite a journey from staff nurse to chief nurse.

I understand PPH is building a "hospital of the future." Tell me about that.

The main hospital is Palomar Medical Center, which is a tertiary medical center; the flagship of our health system. Some of the buildings on this campus are more than 50 years old. The main tower itself is probably pushing 40 by now. When the earthquake hit in Northridge in the 1990s, California state law passed a statute that said all hospitals must meet seismic requirements for earthquake magnitude 7 by the year 2013 and magnitude 8 by 2030. So when we were looking at our options for this campus, we explored whether we should renovate the towers, retrofit them, or build something new on campus. (Our Pomerado campus is seismically sound; however, we need additional capacity so we will be doubling the size of this campus to 210 beds by 2012.). After reviewing the information, we decided to build a new building.

We assembled a steering committee made up of architects, senior leaders, front line staff, nursing, and our visionary CEO, and asked the question, "What do we want to build here?" We were adamant that we didn't want to just build a bigger, more seismically appropriate medical center. When you think about the life of a hospital building itself, it's a 50-year asset. Well, I don't know about you, but I don't know where health care is going be in 2054, but I know it's going to look much different than it does today. And so, we didn't want to build a hospital for today.

We partnered with The Center for Health Design and researched the best ways to provide patient care. We wanted this to be the safest hospital for our patients and we wanted it to be a great place for our staff and physicians. So we assembled champion teams that did the research and came back with recommendations to the senior leadership team for a healthy environment, such as incorporating healing gardens. This building will be spectacular, with trees and conservatories on the 11th floor. You will have access to nature everywhere you go in that building.

But that's just the physical design. We're also implementing a very fundamentally different care delivery model—which is what keeps me awake at night.

I don't know how genomics and the impact of chronicity will affect health care delivery in the more distant future, but we do have a better understanding of what will happen in the short run—say 5 or 10 years. So, in the short run, we have built into this building what we are calling an Interventional Platform, where we are bringing together interventional radiology, cardiology, and the operating room suites all under one umbrella with a contiguous preoperative holding area and post anesthesia care unit.

That's a shift from how hospitals are currently operating. Today, there are 3 distinct areas: interventional radiology, cardiac cath lab, and the operating room, and each department has a separate preop, postop, and recovery area, which is incredibly inefficient. If you think about where surgery is right now and where it will be in the future, it will be minimally invasive and it will rely very heavily on imaging services. And so why not bring them all together and have universal rooms in the Interventional Platform that can be used for cath labs, for ORs, or for interventional radiology?

That is just one innovative design concept here. Our next challenge moving forward is getting the physicians to work together on this concept. I don't think it's going to be as big of an issue for nursing. I believe the challenge for nursing in the future will be what we build in the acuity adaptable care delivery model with the distributed nursing stations.

If you think about what's in the best interest of the patient, then you would never transfer a patient within the hospital. Every time you transfer a patient from one room to another, or one level of acuity to another, you introduce the potential for harm, or medical errors to occur. Every time you hand off a patient, you have the potential for miscommunication. The medications are delayed or may not even be given, and critical things are lost in translation. Maybe the patient's meal doesn't arrive in a timely manner, or we've lost his glasses, hearing aids, or dentures.

The concept here is that all 168 beds in this new hospital will be built to critical care standards, which is the highest level of care you can provide. If a patient needs a critical level of care, he will be admitted to that room, and will not be transferred out of that room when his level of care decreases—instead, the nursing care delivery model changes.

We will be able to provide 1:1 patient care (one nurse to one patient), or 1:2, 1:3, 1:4, 1:5, depending on patient care needs.

Before I go on, I'd like to say that I'm a critical care nurse, and I do not believe that in my career I'm going to get critical care nurses to take care of med/surg patients. That won't happen, and I don't think it should, quite frankly. I do believe though, that nurses will be able to provide critical care to 1 or 2 patients, and if a patient's acuity lessens, then that critical care nurse will be able to adjust his or her patient load in order to provide care for up to 3 patients. The reason I think that is possible, is because we do that today. If you can't transfer patients out of the intensive care unit because the rest of the hospital does not have a bed, then you keep them where they are and provide nursing care accordingly.

This is a fundamental shift in the design of this new hospital, and the nursing care that goes with it. Think about the distance a nurse walks every day in the hospital. It can be between 5 and 7 miles per day. We've designed these patient rooms, which are 320 square feet, so that 80% of what the nurse needs will be at the bedside. We'll have a bedside medication dispensing process, linens, and other supplies. We're also eliminating the central nursing station. Instead, we're having what we call distributed nursing stations. These are small nursing stations built into alcoves outside every patient room. The nurse can look into the patient's room at any time, or turn on the opaque window lighting for privacy.

But where will the team gather to discuss the patient?

We'll have a multi-purpose room on the unit for consultation or multi-disciplinary rounds. We've also designed beautiful lounges on every floor that have access to the gardens.

If you think about it, why does the nursing station exist today? Because that's where the medical record is located. But where is that medical record today and where will it be in the future? It's on your PDA; it's in your palm, right there at your fingertips. At a minimum it's on a tablet that you take in and out of the patient's room. So you don't need a central nurse's station, which is just a hub of activity and noise and chaos. We're bringing as much as we can to the bedside, but we're also keeping a space open for group work, and another for relaxation.

But here's our dilemma. The California Department of Public Health does not recognize the acuity adaptable care delivery model. There's no license category in Title 22 to license that type of bed. They're either licensed "critical care" or they're licensed "med/surg".

I've made it my life's work to change legislation to allow for this model when we open the building in 2011. I don't know how successful this is going to be, but I'm giving it my best shot.

I remember talking about the "hospital of the future" 20 years ago. At the time we believed that technological advancement would minimize the need for extended lengths of stay, while lack of funding would, unfortunately, guarantee shorter hospitalizations and a greater need for home care. We pictured hospitals consisting of the Emergency Department, OR, and critical care units.

That's right. If you really think about what a hospital will look like in the year 2020, I just know it'll be a place where we treat the most critically ill patients.

Are there other hospitals following suit and attempting to redefine the workplace?

Yes there are, and some of them have had more success than others. The most recent one that opened was Dublin Methodist Hospital in Ohio. Apparently their state board has approved an acuity adaptable model of care. There are varying degrees of this model out there, and again, some more successful than others. The downside is trying to maintain the competency of the staff. What I'm doing differently here is having a combination of critical care nurses, intermediate care nurses, and med/surg nurses working together on one unit and assigning them according to patient acuity, rather than hiring all critical care nurses and expecting them to take care of med/surg level patients.

How are you preparing your staff for this transition?

We're implementing pieces and parts of this as we speak. We are piloting a supply distribution process to see how we can bring supplies closer to the staff. We are also moving toward a fully electronic medical record and are piloting wireless tablet devices so our staff will be very comfortable with the whole concept of computer charting. We're even piloting a robot in our ICU to work with our physicians. The physicians make rounds electronically with the robot and do teaching rounds at night with our nursing staff. This robot is amazing! It's stationed in the ICU and the physician logs on from home and can see what's going on in the ICU. You can see what's on the monitors and zoom in and see specific wave forms. You can even see patients' pupil changes.

We see robotics as a real enabler of patient care going forward. This is just the tip of the iceberg.

Are nurses participating in the redesign?

Oh, absolutely. Participation is the name of the game around here. We don't make decisions without the nursing staff and their input into this. Are they all on board? Not all. Some nurses are more techno-savvy than others, but slowly they are coming around to seeing where we need to be. It's just a different way of delivering care. High tech will enable high touch. Mastering the technology will help nurses do what they want to do most, and that is taking care of patients, not taking care of the chart.

I don't think that the technology should drive care, but I do believe that the care process needs to drive how we use technology. Our vision is to provide the safest patient care and be the hospital of the future.

When you talk to people who are interested in entering the profession, how do you describe the nurse of the future?

I speak at the middle school and high school level quite frequently about this. I start by telling them what skills nurses need. If you want to be a nurse you must have compassion. Nothing is going to replace that. No robot in the world is going to sit and hold a patient's hand and comfort them as they are dying. It is just not going to happen. So I don't want to lose sight of that. Critical thinking is extremely important, and for obvious reasons you should be techno-savvy. I also believe the profession needs change agents and historically nursing is not seen that way.

You've accomplished so much in your career, would you consider any of your work to be heroic?

Oh, absolutely not. In my opinion the heroes are my staff. These are the people on the front lines every single day trying to make our nursing vision a reality. My job is to serve them and support them.

We evacuated Pomerado Hospital during the fires in San Diego County in 2007. Do you know who the heroes were? They were the people who came to work while their own homes were on fire and their own families were being evacuated. They came to work. They knew we had to take care of these patients. They're the heroes.

I think what I do takes perseverance, it takes guts, it takes vision, and it takes passion. And I am passionate about what I do.

Lorie K. Shoemaker, RN, MSN, NEA-BC
Chief Nurse Executive
California

CHAPTER 41

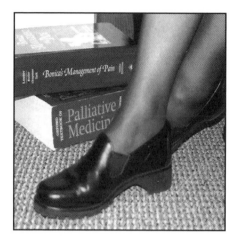

Honor and Opportunity

Throughout the course of one's career, there are opportunities, and there are opportunities taken. I consider myself fortunate to have made good decisions in pursuing my passion in this profession, from working with cancer patients to conducting research and speaking internationally on pain management.

When did you begin to realize that you were drawn to a particular patient population?

I can't recall the exact moment, but over and over in my clinical rotations I loved taking care of oncology patients. In fact, I remember getting chastised by one of my instructors because I was always selecting the most difficult patient. They were almost always the end-stage, septic, cancer patients. When it was time to graduate I chose to stay in oncology.

This is such a complex population—medically, emotionally and spiritually. What inspires you about these patients?

There is so much that I can do as a nurse. I also love the camaraderie amongst cancer patients. They're going through a life and death diagnosis, illness, and treatment. All of a sudden they have a much clearer picture of what this world means and what's important.

I remember taking care of a dying patient at the VA who had a strong family support system. He was in one of the 5-bed wards. The other guys in the room would often help him, but in ways that would never take away from his dignity. They would do it with a joke or a smile.

His wife and daughter were always with him, and it was very clear that he was in his very end stages—he probably had only hours or a day to live. Our typical routine at this stage was to move the person into a private room, and we started to do that until one of the guys pulled me aside and said, "Please don't do that. We know what's happening and we care about him." Now, these were guys with some of the same diagnoses. He continued, "We know his wife and his daughter, and we want to help them. You don't need to move him. Please don't."

That's what I really loved. You could see the most dignified and beautiful aspects of humanity.

Would you consider your work to be heroic?

In some ways I do, because I'm able to really be with a person who is dying. I consider it an honor.

Judith A. Paice, PhD, RN, FAAN
Research Professor of Medicine
Division of Hematology/Oncology
Illinois

CHAPTER 42

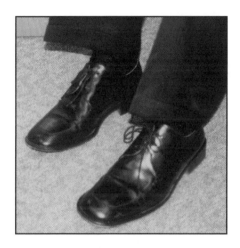

Quality of Life

I was raised by a single woman who was a nurse. My older sister is also a nurse, but her first career was in professional theater and dance. She decided to do something different when her body could no longer support her dream to dance, so at the age of 20 she chose nursing.

Some people find that strange, but my experience is that there is a very creative side to nurses. That creativity is expressed in so many different ways, whether it's caring for someone or developing a budget that can make a difference. There is a creative flair in almost everything that we do.

What led you to management?

I've been a nurse for more than 20 years, and although my background is in critical care, the first management position I accepted was in the ER. The challenge in the ER is that you are dealing with patients and families at very vulnerable stages in their life. In my current role, I work on developing the programmatic aspects of patient care.

How do you do that?

By hiring and developing people, working with physicians, and collaborating on new projects. What gives me the most satisfaction is the fact that I have been able to help individuals develop their careers. That's very rewarding for me.

Is there an experience that stands out for you, in management or at the bedside?

What stands out the most occurred in my first month as a nurse. I was working in a cardiac telemetry unit and was taking care of a gentleman who was a quadriplegic. He had numerous quality of life issues. I remember looking at the patient, but not recognizing his value as an individual. His condition deteriorated throughout the day and he had a cardiac arrest. I remember thinking, "This might be a blessing," but then I turned and saw his wife, and saw how she was responding.

I learned that I was bringing my own values, beliefs, and judgments to the table. I didn't understand the love that they had for one another and the quality of their life together. I grew from that experience. You'd like to think, from a nursing perspective, that you're always giving. This time I was the one who received a gift—one that has stayed with me throughout my career.

Dale E. Beatty, MS, RN
Vice President Patient Services/Chief Nursing Officer
Illinois

CHAPTER 43

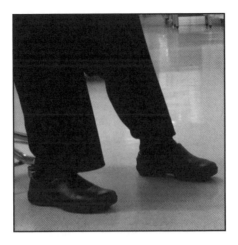

Giving Back

W hen I graduated from college in 1977, women were fighting for their rights and trying to prove themselves in male-dominated professions, but I always wanted to be a nurse. You have power in what you do.

How has the Emergency Department changed over the years?

The improvement in technology alone is amazing, but our consumer has changed as well. We come from an instant gratification society. Patients expect an immediate cure, or quick fix. They'll come in with a stack of papers from the Internet or popular magazines and tell you, "This is what I have. Fix it." Today's consumer is much more educated, but when they self-diagnose, they are also much more dangerous—to themselves.

What we do in the ER is directly related to what our society is like. We're really in the front lines. We've seen so much violence. I think that is what gets to all of us—the shootings, stabbings, and drug-related incidents. I saw what happened when a little girl was used as a human shield in one gang-related incident and was shot dead. I've also comforted a mother who was holding her young son who was a victim of a violent crime.

When a patient comes into the ER he's at his lowest point. We try our hardest to help people not only physically, but psychologically and socially—to get them through that moment. We try our best, and give it our all, with compassion.

I've survived a couple of Chicago Bulls championship winning evenings when the whole city was popping! Ambulances were coming in left and right. People would come in full of blood, and we didn't know if they were shot, stabbed, or hit with a brick. If we can survive 6 Bulls wins, we can survive anything.

How does all this affect you?

I make every day a good day. I enjoy what I do, and I work with great people. That is really what has kept me here.

What is the nicest or the most unexpected thing a patient ever did for you?

Just the other day I had the best experience. A patient walked up to me and said, "I remember you. You were my nurse 7 years ago. You were the only one who listened to me. We talked and talked, and when I came home, I realized just how much you helped me."

Seven years is a long time for someone to remember a conversation. Those are the things that brighten my day. If I can impact one person in any way, that is what is important. That is what gets you going.

I chose to work in this hospital because it's my community hospital. I was born here and I want to give back to the community. It's my home.

Linda Ziarko, RN, BSN
Staff Nurse, Emergency Department
Illinois

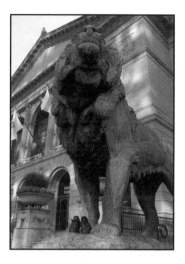

CHAPTER 44

A Place at the Table

"How many of you hold a membership in the symphony? A local museum? The Art Institute?"

That is how I usually start my presentations to nursing groups. The response always surprises me.

I recently presented to the Gerontological Nurse Practitioner Organization in Illinois. They were celebrating their 10th anniversary and I was their dinner speaker. When I asked them how many had subscriptions to the orchestra or museum, a lot of hands went up. That's not true in a lot of places where I've spoken. My topic for the evening was, "Aging, As Depicted in the Arts." The entire presentation is about how the arts can restore the self, and we explore art, music, and poetry.

Following the program they were talking about where they would hold their next meeting and I suggested that they consider the Art Institute or the Chicago Symphony. We had just experienced a program filled with information on the restorative benefits of the arts, and they are thinking about holding their next meeting at a local hospital. Their newly elected president reminded us that the Art Institute would be hosting Edvard Munch's exhibition next year, and we discussed the possibility of having their annual meeting there. Munch is the Norwegian artist who painted The Scream. I had just seen the exhibition elsewhere and loved it. As a matter of fact I use one of his pieces, Death in the Sick-Room, in some of my presentations. Munch does so much in terms of anxiety and depression—his work is somewhat dark—but it also addresses the sanctity of the moment and serves as a wonderful jumping off point for discussion.

I also presented last spring at the Illinois State Convention of the Emergency Nurses Association. There weren't very many hands raised when I asked them about their participation in the arts. At the end of the program I implored them to pick one of the things I had talked about, anything that resonated with them, and make a promise to themselves and to their seat-mate that they would engage in this activity as a way to restore their spirit. There were people there who were so set on learning the latest technology, but were unable to come up with a plan to implement something from the arts in their lives. A nurse approached me and said, "That was a really nice presentation, but I just don't know what I could do right now. I don't think I have the time."

So I have a wide range of responses to this topic of self-care in nursing. I believe in using the arts as a way for nurses to engage in self-care, whether it's using literature, music, or art. The whole idea of restorative space in hospitals or other workplaces is so important.

I wonder if this is simply indicative of our society. Everything is so fast-paced and rushed. We don't have time for anything but work and some family activities. We don't think about replenishing ourselves. What do you recommend?

We need to recognize that we need to help ourselves first. If you don't recognize that, I don't think any amount of program implementation is going to change things. I think that's a significant part of the educational piece of preparing nurses. We emphasize compassion for others; we emphasize empathy. But I don't know that we've ever talked about compassion for ourselves. You know: you've got to put on your own oxygen mask first before you can help someone else.

I think we start off on the right track. I often ask my audiences, "How many of you played a musical instrument as a child?" About three-fourths of the hands in the room go up. I follow that with, "And how many still play an instrument?" Three hands go up. Those things drop out of our lives and they aren't in nursing programs, even in schools that tout the liberal arts. I don't think they're valued. If we let students take a theater course or an art appreciation class, it's seen as frivolous. If they're going to take anything, even at Loyola, we suggest Speech. It's an elective, but we do not encourage a choice among the arts. And yet, any other student who comes to Loyola can choose their electives. Our rationale for recommending Speech is that it's great for leadership or management. We don't place the same value on the arts.

I often wonder why some of our nursing faculty come to teach in a university, when they stay isolated in the school of nursing, or don't do anything with other disciplines. I know the people in the English Department and in Fine Arts. I came here to teach because it's a university and we have so much accessible to us. I know that some of our faculty, who are wonderful scholars in their own right, have never ventured outside their own field. They know everything there is to know about critical care or some other area of nursing, but I believe there's so much more.

I try to teach people to observe more acutely by teaching them to look at art, to notice light and shadow, and other details. It's the idea that you could be informed, in terms of your practice, by Monet and thinking about Impressionism and the impressions we make in walking into a room. Or, appreciating the details of a Caravaggio painting in terms of nursing assessment and diagnosis. When we've taken maternal-child health students on field trips to the Art Institute to look at mothers and babies in art, some of our own colleagues would say, "If you're going on a field trip why wouldn't you go to the history of medicine at the International Museum of Surgical Science?" And that is a great place, but I like to look at Mary Cassatt's paintings of mothers and babies. Or Rafael's Madonna and Child. But that's out of the box thinking. Sadly, I don't think that's universally accepted.

There is a poem I like to read to my nursing audiences. It's entitled "Culpae" and it was written by Carol Battaglia, a recently retired nurse practitioner at our Loyola Medical Center.

Culpae
By Carol Battaglia

Dad, what am I to do?
I'm visiting nursing homes
searching for surrogate
daughters to care for you.

Your needs exceed
what I can provide.
And the oppressive weight
of the guilt I feel
is impossible to hide.

My life affords no space
for you. There's barely
room for me.
So I wander from home to
home hoping to find the
daughter I ought to be.

I hand you over to
waiting arms of strangers
and with this act of final committal,
both of our hearts break
a little.

But dad what am I to do?
I'm trying so hard
to do what is best for you.

Twenty lines. I could be talking about support for people trying to find a placement for their loved one. I could go on and on and give you all the names of the agencies and all the criteria you ought to be looking for. Instead, I'll start with a poem, because I want to engage people and I want them to know what this means to a family. Poetry compresses that.

I had Carol as an RN completion student many years ago and she was given permission in one of her courses to do an alternate assignment. She chose to write some poetry. She had written a few poems before and since then she has published 3 books of poetry that draw upon her experience as a nurse.

We talk a lot in nursing about empathy. Can you really understand another's situation if you haven't had the experience? I think you can, vicariously, through the arts. I think that art is so beautiful by itself, but it can also be so touchingly affective. I take nurses and students on educational tours throughout France and Italy, and they are always touched by actually seeing Michelangelo's Pieta in Rome. They've heard about it, they've seen pictures of it—but to actually see it is amazing.

On the other hand, I had a student once who lost her daughter in a terrible automobile accident 2 years before. When she saw the Pieta she said, "Oh my God. Michelangelo never lost a child or he wouldn't have made Mary look so serene." What a poignant discussion you can have using both observations.

We first met while I was working on a federally funded Nurse Retention Grant, and you were working on developing a restorative space for nursing at the same hospital. The topic of restorative space is very popular, but I find that nurses can barely leave the unit to enjoy a Nurses Week celebration activity.

But again, isn't that self-care? Isn't it self-care, or lack of self-care, when nurses don't go to lunch? The idea of a restorative space came out of a series of overnight retreats we had for the nurse managers in that hospital system. We focused on the four elements in addressing self-care: water (emotion), air (breath), earth (food), and fire (creativity). We chose to work with the nurse managers because we felt they were pivotal people in terms of creating change at their hospitals. During those retreats, we used music, art, and poetry related to the elements, and out of those retreats every hospital's group of managers acknowledged a need for restorative space.

We found that in terms of self-care, nurses don't eat lunch—or they eat lunch in the dirty utility room, or at their desks. We worked with the nurses to plan for a healthier lunch once they returned to work. At least once a week these participants would have to meet for lunch in the cafeteria. Granted, some of those cafeterias weren't very nice places. Some didn't have any windows, and overall they weren't very relaxing places, but at least they would leave their desks and work environments for a few moments of self-care. We were just talking about doing lunch, not even savoring lunch. Savoring just wasn't in their vocabulary.

The other issue we tackled surrounded drinking water. You'll hear nurses say, "If I drink water then I have to go to the bathroom, and I don't have time to go to the bathroom." So if you don't drink water you get urinary tract infections!

Do you think physicians go without lunch? You think top level administrators go without lunch? They often go out to dine at a restaurant or the local country club. Why do nurses think they don't deserve lunch? We also tell nurses that they can't go on a break until they get all of their work done. Do you think people working in offices don't take a break? I'm thinking, "Hail to the smokers." At least they're getting out.

And then I started to think about our own faculty and about the students they take to the units. "Listen," they whisper, "if we don't eat lunch we can get out of here sooner. Instead of 3pm, we'll get out at 2pm." And look what happens—now we're actually teaching poor self-care.

We planned an activity during the retreat for the nurses to create a place for themselves at the table. It was an arts and crafts event, and of course everyone was rolling their eyes, but everyone had to make place mats that they brought to the dinner.

Dinner was a special event. They were given a letter prior to attending, asking them to bring something special to wear. They also had to talk about the item they brought and why they felt it represented them. The nurses from one of the hospitals in the system brought tiaras. It's so interesting that that's how the nurses think of themselves at that hospital. Tiaras! We also asked them to bring something of meaning from either their home or office.

Then we focused on enjoying the dinner; savoring the food. We placed special emphasis on breaking the bread, and pouring the wine. People were commenting however, that they couldn't remember sitting down for a meal with their own families lately. It was very moving. We called this exercise, Coming to the Table.

Of course, this is a metaphor for being part of the decision-making process at the hospital or in the community. Be at the table. This is where decisions are being made. Creating a place for yourself at the table is so important, and you'll never be at the table if you don't take the responsibility for creating that place. The table is also a place to share nourishment and socialize and we should make ourselves available for both.

How do you recommend we do that—as individuals and as a profession?

You have to believe you deserve a place at the table. I think that we deserve a place, but I think that the majority of nurses do not think so. I think there are nursing leaders who obviously do think so, and have broken the glass ceiling, but the majority of nurses who come to this profession choose a subordinate role, or they are squashed in the process. I know that there are faculty who aren't really thrilled with certain assertive students and squash them at every opportunity. And if the students had any feelings of power or strength they are told to keep in their place.

I don't know that we adequately address power and leadership in management courses for undergrads. They can hardly think about being a delegator because they've always been a delegate. And even at the graduate level, I'm not sure if we talk enough about the long-term career paths in nursing or leadership opportunities you ought to be looking for.

We address all nursing career options in school, but what are those options? They're med/surg, ortho, psych, maternal-child, etc. "Isn't it wonderful?" we say to the students. "We have this array of options." But we're limiting them.

Several years ago we celebrated our 45th class reunion from Loyola University. We recalled that in 1960, baccalaureate nursing education was relatively new, and we were labeled by some as snobby, but we had been told by the faculty that, as a class, we could do anything. Opportunity favors the prepared. In my own career I have tried to do my homework and I asked questions. If you don't know something about a financial statement, ask what that line's about. I'd ask a lot of questions and all of a sudden I was the Chair of the Lutheran General Board, and then I was the Chair of the Advocate Health Care Board. It doesn't happen by chance. I think it's a combination of being prepared and also knowing you have a contribution to make that will be unique.

How can we set a place at the table for our profession?

We need the self-recognition to know that we belong at the table. And I think we need to seek a mentor to help us see where the table is, and what implements/tools we'll need. To take the metaphor further....we should ask ourselves if we'd like to be at the head of the table or be a diner? Do we want to make the decisions, or simply participate in the process? I don't think every opportunity must be located within the INA (Illinois Nurses Association), the ANA (American Nurses Association), or the NLN (National League for Nursing). I think they're in other places, certainly in terms of the Illinois Board of Registration and Regulation. Who's going to be there at the table to make decisions and be articulate enough or assertive enough to let nursing be heard well? It was surprising that we were one of the last states to get prescriptive powers for advanced practice nurses. I think there are all kinds of tables where nurses can make a unique contribution because of the background that they bring.

We're probably not very media savvy. We ought to have a greater presence in newspapers and magazines. We ought to be publishing in *Family Circle*. The checkout counter is where people get their image of nursing. In fact, I mentioned this idea to a colleague who needs 3 more publications to go for full professor. I suggested that she publish something in *Family Circle*. It certainly would not get her promoted, but it would get nursing noticed.

I also think it is interesting to see the types of thank you's nurses receive from their grateful patients. Many times it's a box of candy or a vase of flowers. Doctors receive an endowed chair. Where is the endowed chair in our thank you?

The Niehoff School of Nursing was named for Conrad and Marcella Niehoff, who were in the automotive business. When the announcement was made that 4 million dollars was coming to Loyola's School of Nursing, people were amazed. That was a significant amount of money 25 years ago. But the story from Mrs. Niehoff was that her husband was so well cared for by nurses that not to do this would be an insult to his memory.

I know that there are more endowed chairs in nursing schools today. It's often initiated, however, by development office staff who try to find out a little about nursing and then identify potential donors that might be a good fit, rather than building on an experience the patient/donor had with a nurse.

In keeping with the title of the book, do you consider your work to be heroic?

I consider this work to be groundbreaking, and I'm saving lives every day. Two nurses approached me after a Nurses Week presentation last year and said, "You know, the girl sitting next to me is my best friend and we're going to leave here today and buy season opera tickets." I'm saving lives, enhancing lives, enriching lives. I talk about taking our rightful place at the larger table, but I think we also need to prepare ourselves to ask for a table for two.

Mary Ann McDermott, RN, EdD, FAAN
Professor Emerita
Illinois

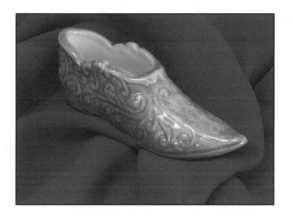

Afterword

I believe in serendipity. I've encountered too many surprising, happy coincidences while writing this book to attribute it all to chance. Most of the nurses I interviewed (other than close friends and family) were introduced to me under the most interesting circumstances. My hairstylist suggested that I interview his mother because her work as a nurse impressed him so much while he was growing up (Francine Gust). The gallery owner of my first exhibition informed me that his college roommate became a mental health nurse, and he married a nurse as well (Ed and Noreen Shilney). A nurse who attended one of my keynotes asked me why I didn't have any combat boots from nurses in the military, and gave me his son's contact information in Iraq (Sam Matta). I interviewed the father as well (Chad Matta).

One of the most recent of these serendipitous encounters occurred online. I was putting the finishing touches on the last of the stories when I took a break and went window shopping on eBay. I found a beautiful little porcelain shoe with scroll work that resembled my logo. When I read the description, I was struck by the seller's story. Very simply, he wrote that the piece was a German antique, and he knew that because he bought it for his mother while he was stationed in Germany during the Vietnam War. He bought it from a woman who needed money for groceries. She wouldn't accept a handout and insisted that this soldier take the heirloom.

This was Veteran's Day, and I was moved to buy the little shoe. In my note to the seller I commented on the story and thanked him for serving. He wrote back saying he appreciated my comment. He went on to tell me a little more about his experience coming home after the war. "It wasn't pleasant," he told me. "Sorry. I never do this," he wrote. "Something made me want to tell you these few things."

I don't engage in long letter-writing to eBay sellers either, but there was a genuineness about this gentleman, and I wrote another message back. I thanked him for sharing his story with me and shared with him why I was buying his shoe. I told him that I was a nurse and that I had interviewed nurses from across the country and in the military, and the stories would be published in this book. I thanked him again for sharing the provenance of my purchase.

His note back to me brought tears to my eyes. It's best to let his letter speak for itself:

> **"What an awesome thing you're doing. My wife was a cancer nurse and dialysis nurse, then she lost her sight. Did you know, she had to take her brother home from the hospital after his amputation, just to correct his sugar levels? Amazing. Stats say that hospitals kill more of these patients each year. And it isn't the nurses. They do what they are told. What happened?"**

He sent that message to me as I was finishing Karen Thomas' story, *Open Heart*. In exchange for his candor, I decided to send him the last few paragraphs of her story. It was uncanny how his note dovetailed with what I was editing.

Shortly after sending my message, I received another e-mail. This time he added his comments throughout the excerpt from Karen Thomas' *Open Heart*:

Health care is going through tremendous changes. Where do you see the future of our profession?

We have a young staff on our unit, and I told them that in 5 years I want them to be a team that is cohesive and strong, because let's face it, I'm likely to be their patient in another 4 or 5 years. I want them to be powerful diagnostically, powerful therapeutically, and powerful spiritually, to treat a person like myself who wants the same level of care that I would give to any one of them were our roles reversed.

Comment: Amen to that.

I've noticed a trend recently that some young nurses push themselves into a master's program so quickly that they rush in with only a year or two of nursing experience under their belts. They start working toward becoming an advance practice nurse and I think they confuse having a Master's in nursing with being a masterful nurse.

Comment: And a HUGE Amen to that!

I also think we should have an almost evangelical spirit in terms of insisting that this next generation is qualified to serve on every level. We're graduating nurses right, left, and center who come out with enough general knowledge to pass the NCLEX exam, but we have lost a lot of the humanizing elements having a generation largely raised without the humanities. How many students today have any sense of literature, philosophy, or the arts that teach us so much about the human spirit?

Comment: And there lies the problem!

We have lost much of that within American popular culture. It is time to pull ourselves back to the center as a nation.

I'd like to tell nurses just entering the field to slow down and really absorb the gestalt of nursing. As a novice nurse, you might be able to speak the language, but you don't have the naturalness of someone who is fluent. That takes time and years of practice. I'll sometimes ask a new nurse if they play a musical instrument. Take the piano, for instance. Do you remember the first time you ever sat on the bench looking at the keys, then looking at the music and back again at the keys? How were you about your fourth year? You probably weren't even looking at the keys anymore. Nursing is a lot like that. As a new nurse you're going to be looking at every step in order to complete the tasks at hand. Performing the skills of nursing is going to take all of your energy. The art of nursing will come later.

You've mentioned both the art and the science of nursing. Would you consider your work as a nurse to be heroic?

Oh, absolutely! Both of my brothers are physicians and they have both said to me, "Nurses are really the heart of medicine, aren't they?"

Comment: In my humble opinion, they sure used to be.

I believe we truly are.

You can be a proficient nurse in terms of getting the medication to the bedside in a timely manner and completing all of your charting, but when it comes to being a true healer, that's a different matter altogether. We give patients back their dignity in so many ways and we find that gentle moment to help them reconnect with themselves.

Comment: This is what they should be able to do, however, [there is] no time for the gentle moment, or to connect, really connect with their patient. I've seen so much lack of patience....it breaks your heart.

We give patients the courage to heal.

Comment: Well, my wife sure did. In fact there are many families and doctors alike that have said to her, "You loved them into living 5 more years, 2 more years, etc." And she did. She saw the patient, but she also made sure to see the human being. She saw the woman, behind just being the mom, and the man behind just being the dad. The stages are basically the same for the pronounced terminal, however a good nurse can give them the gift of love in their own minds, that they do matter....I could go on but she could explain it better. Don't need to though, because you know. God bless you, really bless you with this. Tom ✍

I took on this project in 2001 because we were starting to experience a nursing shortage unparalleled in our history, and rather than reading about what we could do to alleviate the problem, I read inflammatory stories in major newspapers and magazines that pointed the finger at nurses. Our mistakes, I read, were contributing to poor patient outcomes. More specifically, the headline in the *Chicago Tribune* read: "Nursing Mistakes Kill/Injure Thousands." It's true that our numbers are dwindling at the bedside, but what is causing this? I felt we needed a public rebuttal, and that is how this book was born.

Tom's right. Something has changed in health care, but there are still enough intelligent, passionate, caring nurses in all age groups who make a difference in patients' lives every day. I hope this book will offer them a voice in a very public way. Every time I mention my work, I hear stories about mothers, sisters, uncles, and neighbors who are nurses and who "should be in this book." I welcome all of their stories.

America's nurses are telling their stories and I encourage you to join in the discussion. Write to me and tell me your quiet victories, your challenges and your ideas. Better yet, share your stories at work, with your neighbors, your local papers, and favorite blogs.

I believe it's time for nurses to take their rightful place at the table and participate in the discussions affecting the future of health care and of our profession. Please join me.

www.irenestemler.com
www.slackbooks.com

Irene Stemler, RN, BSN

WAIT
...*There's More!*

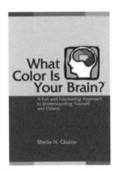

What Color Is Your Brain? A Fun and Fascinating Approach to Understanding Yourself and Others
Sheila N. Glazov
176 pp, Soft Cover, 2008, ISBN 13: 978-1-55642-807-4, Order# 88073, **$16.95**

Enjoyable, insightful, and easy-to-read, *What Color Is Your Brain?* is a guide to exploring who we are, why others see us the way they do, and how the four "brain colors" or personality types play a role in our everyday lives.

Written for readers of all ages, genders, and backgrounds, this book is intended to facilitate effective communication and cooperation while minimizing frustration in numerous aspects of our everyday lives—at work and home, in dating and marital relationships, with team projects, among family members and friends, and within a mixture of other interpersonal connections. *What Color Is Your Brain?* is a guide to exploring who we are, why others see us the way they do, and how the four "brain colors" or personality types play a role in our everyday lives.

"I highly recommend this book as an enlightening, fun-filled guide to learning more about yourself and others."

—Aida J. Sapp, PhD, APRN, BC, LMFT, *Associate Professor, College of Nursing, The University of Mary Hardin-Baylor, Belton, Texas*

Please visit

www.slackbooks.com
to order any of these titles!
24 Hours a Day...7 Days a Week!

Attention Industry Partners!

Whether you are interested in buying multiple copies of a book, chapter reprints, or looking for something new and different— we are able to accommodate your needs.

Multiple Copies

At attractive discounts starting for purchases as low as 25 copies for a single title, SLACK Incorporated will be able to meet all of your needs.

Chapter Reprints

SLACK Incorporated is able to offer the chapters you want in a format that will lead to success. Bound with an attractive cover, use the chapters that are a fit specifically for your company. Available for quantities of 100 or more.

Customize

SLACK Incorporated is able to create a specialized custom version of any of our products specifically for your company.

Please contact the Marketing Communications Director of Health Care Books and Journals for further details on multiple copy purchases, chapter reprints or custom printing at 1-800-257-8290 or 1-856-848-1000.

*Please note all conditions are subject to change.

CODE: 328

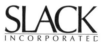

SLACK Incorporated • Health Care Books and Journals
6900 Grove Road • Thorofare, NJ 08086

1-800-257-8290 or 1-856-848-1000

Fax: 1-856-848-6091 • E-mail: orders@slackinc.com • Visit: www.slackbooks.com